ELECTRON SPIN RESONANCE
IN SEMICONDUCTORS

MONOGRAPHS ON ELECTRON SPIN RESONANCE

Editor: H. M. Assenheim, Hilger & Watts Ltd., London, England

Electron Spin Resonance
in
Semiconductors

G. LANCASTER

University of Keele
Keele, England

PLENUM PRESS
NEW YORK
1967

Published in the U.S.A. by
PLENUM PRESS
a division of
PLENUM PUBLISHING CORPORATION
227 West 17th Street, New York, New York 10011

Library of Congress Catalog Card No. 67-21450

First published by
Hilger & Watts Ltd.

Printed in Great Britain by J. W. Arrowsmith Ltd., Bristol

703609

EDITOR'S PREFACE

Since the study of the solid state began it has been necessary to use increasingly refined experimental techniques, of which electron spin resonance is an important example, in the effort to gain information concerning the structure and properties of an immense and varied range of solids. In the last two decades the great commercial demand for solid-state electronic devices has stimulated research into the fundamental properties of semiconductors.

At the same time as semiconductor devices were becoming technologically important, the technique of electron spin resonance was first being used on a large scale, principally at the Clarendon Laboratory, Oxford.

Both solid-state physics and electron spin resonance have now reached the stage where they are useful to each other, primarily in the realm of the atomic properties of matter.

Dr Lancaster's book is one of a series of monographs that aims at covering as comprehensively as possible the field of electron spin resonance. His book has been written for those who wish to know something about the way in which the electron spin resonance technique has been used in the study of semiconductors. It also has value for specialists who may need an authoritative work of reference, and for workers in allied subjects who wish to use this technique to further their work. Much of his treatise deals with electron spin resonance in crystals of silicon and germanium containing specific impurities, as these materials are of greatest interest. Practical results are discussed wherever possible.

H. M. ASSENHEIM

PREFACE

The greatest interest shown in semiconducting materials reflects both their technological importance and their great usefulness as model solids because of their high purity and relatively simple crystal structure.

Throughout this text the general aim is to assist those unfamiliar with semiconductors or electron spin resonance, or both, to gain an insight into the vast amount of research work which has been carried out in this field. To this end analytical mathematical proofs have been largely omitted and results of physical significance with regard to semiconductors rather than to the theory of electron spin resonance have been emphasized.

I should like to acknowledge the assistance I have received from many workers in this field who have permitted me to reproduce their published and unpublished results. The bibliography is intended to be exhaustive but I should like to take this opportunity of apologizing in advance for any omissions I may have made.

Finally, I should like to thank my wife and Mrs. E. M. Brookes for their secretarial assistance in the preparation of this book.

G. LANCASTER
UNIVERSITY OF KEELE
January, 1966

CONTENTS

Chapter 1

Energy Bands and Impurity States in Semiconductors

SEMICONDUCTORS

The term 'semiconductor' is used to describe a large number of materials whose electrical conductivities lie between those of insulators ($\sim 10^{-10}$ mho/cm or less) and metals ($\sim 10^5$ mho/cm).

In a metal either the highest occupied energy band is only partly filled with electrons (e.g. the alkali metals) or else two energy bands overlap so that there are unoccupied electron states in both bands (e.g. the divalent metals).[1] Thus, in both cases, there are electrons present, in large numbers, which are free to move under the influence of externally applied fields, giving rise to high electrical conductivities.

If the highest occupied energy band is completely filled with electrons, then the material is an insulator. In semiconductors the energy-band structure is essentially the same as that in insulators, except that electrons can be introduced into the conduction band, or free holes into the valence band, in small, but significant, numbers. As the free-charge carriers are usually produced by thermal excitation across an energy gap, semiconductors can be characterized by a negative temperature coefficient of resistance, although there are exceptions to this rule, depending on the concentration and type of added impurity, and on the temperature.

Silicon carbide, graphite, and the Group II–VI compounds are often classed as semiconductors, but, in this text, discussion will be restricted to the elemental semiconductors belonging to Group IV of the Periodic Table and to the Group III–V compounds.[2] There is also a large class of organic compounds which exhibit semiconducting properties,[3] but they will not be considered here.

§1.2

ELECTRON SPIN RESONANCE

In principle, electron spin resonance (E.S.R.) may be observed in any system that has unpaired electrons,[4] and many such systems are found in semiconductors.

The only unpaired-electron system present in intrinsic semiconductors is that of the conduction electrons. However, practical difficulties, such as the relatively small number of conduction electrons and short spin-lattice relaxation times, preclude their observation by the E.S.R. technique.

In fact, E.S.R. has only been observed in extrinsic semiconductors and the systems which have been investigated may, at this early stage, be grouped under five headings.

(*a*) 'Shallow' donor and acceptor impurities
(*b*) 'Deep' impurities
(*c*) Conduction electrons
(*d*) Radiation-damage centres
(*e*) Surface states

E.S.R. was first observed in a semiconductor by England and Schneider[5] when investigating manganese as an impurity in ZnS. Portis *et al.*[6] were the first to report E.S.R. in a Group IV semiconductor. The resonance line in *n*-type silicon was observed over a wide range of temperature and attributed to conduction electrons. Fletcher *et al.*[7] first noticed E.S.R. for electrons bound to shallow donor impurities in silicon. Since then semiconductors have been the subject of intensive research using the E.S.R. technique.

One very important result of the great strides made in semiconductor technology is that extremely high purity materials (e.g. electrically active impurities $< 10^{12} \, cm^{-3}$ in silicon) have become available. Such materials, especially when they have a relatively simple crystal structure as the semiconductors mentioned in §1.1, are extremely useful model solids. The E.S.R. spectra obtained from these solids, which are characterized by tetrahedral symmetry of the lattice sites and predominantly covalent bonding, have been compared with those obtained in predominantly ionic solids. In this way, the effect of covalent bonding has been observed on such parameters of the E.S.R. spectrum as the *g*-value, the zero field splitting coefficient and the hyperfine interaction constant. The hyperfine interaction with magnetic isotopes of the host crystal has enabled the unpaired electron wave function to be evaluated at neighbouring lattice sites.

§1.3

SHALLOW DONOR STATES IN SILICON AND GERMANIUM

Shallow impurity states in general are of vital importance in the control of the electrical properties of semiconductors, and the E.S.R. technique has made a large contribution towards the elucidation of their structure. Hence, it is worthwhile examining in some detail the physical description of these states, particularly in silicon and germanium in which they are now very well understood.

In a single crystal of pure material, the Schroedinger equation for a single electron is

$$\left(-\frac{\hbar^2}{2m_e}\nabla^2 + V\right)\psi = E\psi \qquad (1.1)$$

where V is the periodic crystalline potential. This equation can be rewritten as

$$-\frac{\hbar^2}{2m^*}\nabla^2\psi = E\psi \qquad (1.2)$$

where m^* is the effective mass of the electron. Now consider the effect of adding Group V atoms, which enter the lattice as substitutional impurities. Four electrons are used to satisfy the tetrahedral bonding at a lattice site (see Fig. 1.1). The fifth (donor electron) is unpaired and thus the neutral impurity centre is paramagnetic. As we shall see, the ground state of this centre lies slightly below the conduction-band edge (~ 0.045 eV). Hence the donor electron is easily excited into the conduction band and the resulting ionized centre is non-paramagnetic. The Hamiltonian for this electron is $(-\hbar^2/2m^*\nabla^2 + \mathcal{U})$, where $\mathcal{U}(= e^2/\epsilon r)$ is the additional potential due to the impurity atom. r is the distance of the donor electron from the donor nucleus and ϵ is the dielectric constant of the medium ($\epsilon = 12$ and 16 for silicon and germanium respectively).

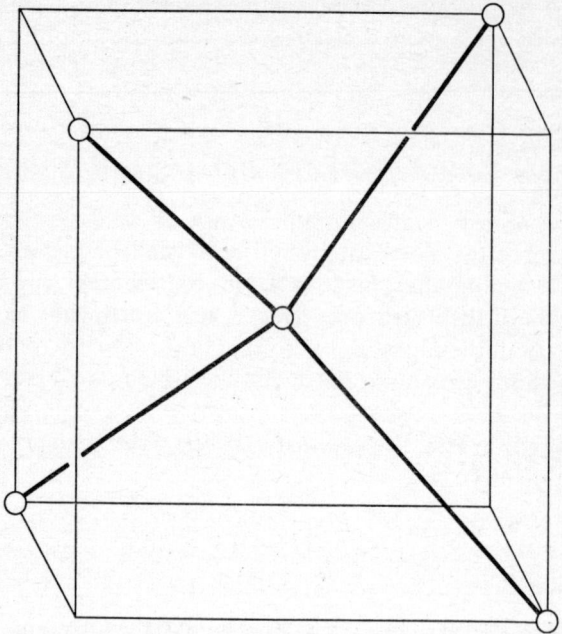

FIG. 1.1. Tetrahedral bonding. Each atom is linked to four nearest neighbours situated at the corners of a regular tetrahedron.

The Schroedinger equation now becomes

$$\left(-\frac{\hbar^2}{2m^*}\nabla^2 + \mathscr{U}\right)\chi = E\chi \tag{1.3}$$

This equation is conveniently solved by using Wannier[8] functions $a_n(\mathbf{r}-\mathbf{l})$, where n is a band index and $\mathbf{l}$ is the vector to a lattice site. The Wannier functions are defined through

$$\psi_{n,\mathbf{k}}(\mathbf{r}) = \frac{1}{\sqrt{N}} \sum_{\mathbf{l}} \exp(i\mathbf{k}.\mathbf{l})a_n(\mathbf{r}-\mathbf{l}) \tag{1.4}$$

Here $\psi_{n,\mathbf{k}}(\mathbf{r})$ is the true Bloch function in the nth band. Alternatively

$$a_n(\mathbf{r}-\mathbf{l}) = \frac{1}{\sqrt{N}} \sum_{\mathbf{k}} \exp(-i\mathbf{k}.\mathbf{l})\psi_{n,\mathbf{k}}(\mathbf{r}) \tag{1.5}$$

If a solution to equation (1.3) takes the form

$$\chi(\mathbf{r}) = \sum_{n,1} F_n(\mathbf{l})a_n(\mathbf{r}-\mathbf{l}) \tag{1.6}$$

then an equation akin to a Schroedinger equation is obtained (see Appendix):

$$[E(-i\nabla)+\mathscr{U}]F_n(\mathbf{l}) = EF_n(\mathbf{l}) \tag{1.7}$$

which is evaluated at each lattice site. Here it should be remembered that $\mathbf{k}_{op} = -i\nabla$. In obtaining this equation it has been assumed that $\mathscr{U}$ varies slowly from lattice site to lattice site so that inter-band matrix elements such as $\langle a_{n'}{}^*(\mathbf{r}-\mathbf{l}')|\mathscr{U}|a_n(\mathbf{r}-\mathbf{l})\rangle$ can be neglected. The assumption also means that

$$\langle a_n{}^*(\mathbf{r}-\mathbf{l}')|\mathscr{U}|a_n(\mathbf{r}-\mathbf{l})\rangle = U\delta_{ll'}$$

where $\delta_{ll'} = 0$ for $l \neq l'$ and 1 for $l = l'$ because of the orthogonality of Wannier functions on different lattice sites. We shall see that the assumption concerning the slowly varying nature of $\mathscr{U}$ breaks down near the impurity nucleus. It is natural to interpolate between lattice sites and treat $F_n(\mathbf{l})$ as a continuous function.

From equation (1.7) we see that $F(\mathbf{r})$ (the band index has been dropped since we are concerned now with only a single band) satisfies a hydrogen-like so-called effective mass equation where $(-\hbar^2/2m^*)\nabla^2$ has been replaced by an equivalent Hamiltonian $E(-i\nabla)$. Hence the total electron wave function at a lattice site is given by

$$\chi = F(\mathbf{r})\sum_{\mathbf{k}} \exp(i\mathbf{k}.\mathbf{r}).u_{\mathbf{k}}(\mathbf{r}) \tag{1.8}$$

A characteristic of silicon and germanium is that the minima of their conduction bands do not lie at the centre of the Brillouin zone in the reduced zone scheme[9,10] (see Fig. 1.2). In silicon the minima ('valleys') lie along the $\langle 100\rangle$ directions in reciprocal space and are situated 85 per cent of the way from the centre to the boundary of the zone. Thus there are six equivalent minima. In germanium the minima are situated at the boundary of the zone in the $\langle 111\rangle$ directions and hence there are four equivalent minima. Near the conduction-band minima the equi-energy surfaces are ellipsoids of revolution about the directions in which the

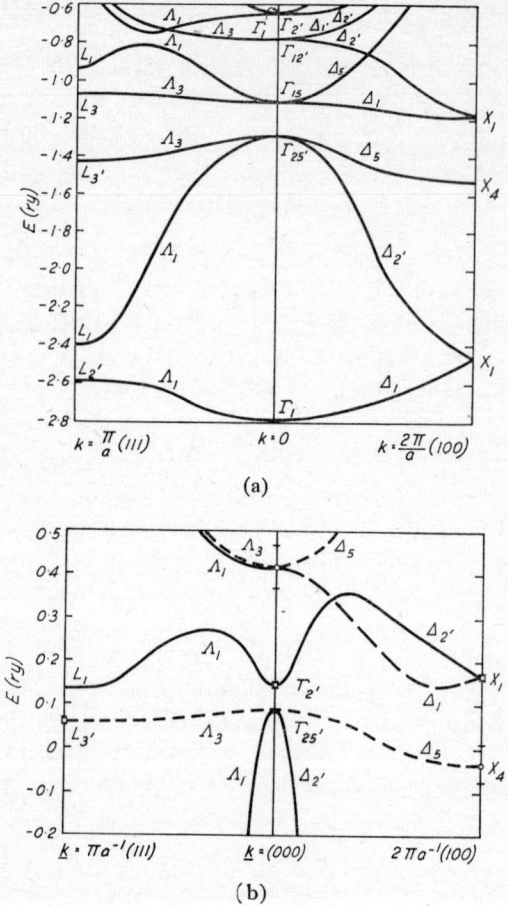

(a)

(b)

Fig. 1.2. Energy-band structures in silicon and germanium.
(a) Silicon (after Kleinman and Phillips[9]): The conduction band is denoted by Δ_1 and Λ_3 in the [100] and [111] directions respectively, and the minimum occurs 85 per cent of the way from Γ_{15} to X_1.
(b) Germanium (after Phillips[10]): The conduction band is denoted by Λ_1, and $\Delta_{2'}$ in the [111] and [100] directions respectively, the lowest minimum occurring at the point L_1.

minima lie, and in silicon, for example, are specified by

$$\frac{\hbar^2}{2m_{\parallel}}(k_z-k_0)^2+\frac{\hbar^2}{2m_{\perp}}(k_x^2+k_y^2)=E \qquad (1.9)$$

where the z-axis coincides with one of the $\langle 100 \rangle$ axes and k_0 is the value of k at which the minimum occurs. It should also be noted that the two components of the tensor for the effective mass perpendicular to the axis of the ellipsoid are equal, being different from the component parallel to the axis of the ellipsoid.

As we are going to be concerned only with states near the conduction-band minimum, equation (1.8) is approximated by[11]

$$\chi = F(\mathbf{r})\psi(\mathbf{k}_0, \mathbf{r}) \tag{1.10}$$

If the effective mass were isotropic, then the $F(\mathbf{r})$ would simply be hydrogen-like wave functions, e.g. for the ground state

$$F(\mathbf{r}) = \frac{1}{(\pi a^{*3})^{1/2}} \cdot \exp(-r/a^*) \tag{1.11}$$

where the effective Bohr radius is given by

$$a^* = \frac{\hbar^2 \epsilon}{e^2 m^*} \tag{1.12}$$

and the energy level spectrum would be given by

$$E_n = \frac{1}{n^2} \frac{m^* e^4}{2\epsilon^2 \hbar^2} \qquad n = 1, 2, \ldots \tag{1.13}$$

Since the $\psi(\mathbf{k}_0, \mathbf{r})$ in equation (1.10) can be chosen from j equivalent conduction-band minima, the donor levels given by equation (1.13) are j-fold degenerate. However, near the donor-impurity nucleus, the foregoing arguments break down since in the assumed form of $\mathscr{U}(\mathbf{r})$ the macroscopic dielectric constant is used. At distances of the order of a few inter-atomic spacings, the concept of a dielectric constant is meaningless and the Hamiltonian has to be modified. The true Hamiltonian must be invariant under the tetrahedral symmetry group T_d and the j-fold degeneracy is partially lifted. Thus the wave functions describing the donor states are written in the form

$$\Psi^{(i)} = \sum_j \alpha_j^{(i)} \chi_j \tag{1.14}$$

where

$$\chi_j = F_j(\mathbf{r})\psi_j(\mathbf{k}_0, \mathbf{r}) \tag{1.15}$$

and the $\alpha_j{}^{(i)}$ are numerical coefficients specifying the combinations of the χ_j function. Group theoretical considerations yield the following linear combinations corresponding to the various irreducible representations of T_d:[12,13]

Silicon

$$\text{Singlet} \quad \alpha_j^{(1)} = \frac{1}{\sqrt{6}}(1, 1, 1, 1, 1, 1)$$

$$\text{Doublet}\begin{cases} \alpha_j^{(2)} = \dfrac{1}{\sqrt{12}}(1, 1, 1, 1, -2, -2) \\[3mm] \alpha_j^{(3)} = \dfrac{1}{2}(1, 1, -1, -1, 0, 0) \end{cases}$$

$$\text{Triplet}\begin{cases} \alpha_j^{(4)} = \dfrac{1}{\sqrt{2}}(1, -1, 0, 0, 0, 0) \\[3mm] \alpha_j^{(5)} = \dfrac{1}{\sqrt{2}}(0, 0, 1, -1, 0, 0) \\[3mm] \alpha_j^{(6)} = \dfrac{1}{\sqrt{2}}(0, 0, 0, 0, 1, -1) \end{cases} \qquad (1.16)$$

Germanium

$$\text{Singlet} \quad \alpha_j^{(1)} = \frac{1}{2}(1, 1, 1, 1)$$

$$\text{Triplet}\begin{cases} \alpha_j^{(2)} = \dfrac{1}{2}(1, 1, -1, -1) \\[3mm] \alpha_j^{(3)} = \dfrac{1}{\sqrt{2}}(1, -1, 0, 0) \\[3mm] \alpha_j^{(4)} = \dfrac{1}{\sqrt{2}}(0, 0, 1, -1) \end{cases} \qquad (1.17)$$

These considerations alone do not allow us to predict which of the groups of states lies lowest.

To take account of the anisotropic effective mass, Kohn[11] assumed a simple variational envelope function for the donor ground state of the form

$$F = \frac{1}{(\pi a^2 b)^{1/2}} \cdot \exp\{-[(x^2+y^2)/a^2 + z^2/b^2]^{1/2}\} \qquad (1.18)$$

and found

$$a_{\text{Si}} = 25 \cdot 0 \times 10^{-8} \text{ cm} \qquad b_{\text{Si}} = 14 \cdot 2 \times 10^{-8} \text{ cm}$$
$$a_{\text{Ge}} = 64 \cdot 5 \times 10^{-8} \text{ cm} \qquad b_{\text{Ge}} = 22 \cdot 7 \times 10^{-8} \text{ cm} \qquad (1.19)$$

Thus we see that the wave function is not spherical but is compressed in the direction of the axis of the ellipsoidal equi-energy surface. Over distances of a few lattice spacings the electron can be effectively thought of as being in a Bloch state, but over distances of the order of a^* the Bloch wave is modulated appreciably by the

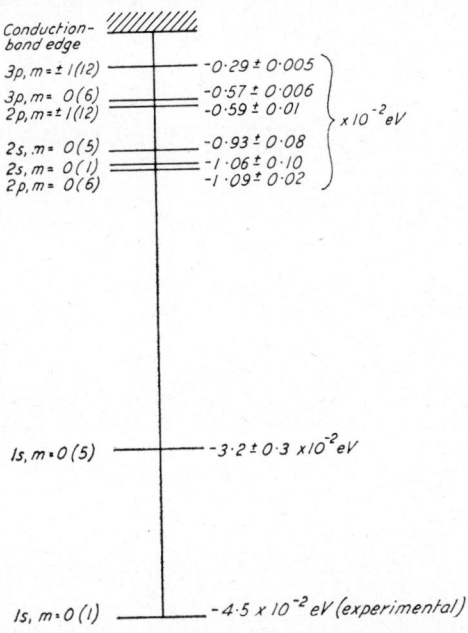

Fig. 1.3. A theoretical spectrum of energy levels for a phosphorus atom in silicon. The numbers in parentheses refer to the number of (approximately) degenerate states, spin degeneracy not included.

(By courtesy of W. Kohn[11] and Academic Press Inc.)

envelope function $F(\mathbf{r})$. The theoretical spectrum of energy levels for phosphorus in silicon is shown in Fig. 1.3.

E.S.R. experiments on electrons bound to donor-impurity atoms in silicon and germanium show well-resolved isotropic hyperfine interaction,[14] owing to the magnetic moments of the donor nuclei. This is a clear indication that the singlet state lies lowest, since isotropic hyperfine interaction is proportional to $|\Psi(\text{o})|^2$, and of the states represented in (1.16) and (1.17), only the singlets have $|\Psi(\text{o})|^2 \neq \text{o}$.

The value for $|\Psi(\text{o})|^2$ calculated from the foregoing theory was about ten times smaller than the value obtained from the measured hyperfine interactions. This discrepancy was removed when the measured values for the donor-impurity ionization energy were substituted into

$$-\frac{\hbar^2}{2m_\parallel}\frac{\partial^2 F}{\partial z^2} - \frac{\hbar^2}{2m_\perp}\left(\frac{\partial^2 F}{\partial x^2} + \frac{\partial^2 F}{\partial y^2}\right) + \mathscr{U}F = EF \qquad (1.20)$$

and new wave functions calculated. The modified wave functions are more 'peaked' around the donor-impurity nucleus and the values for $|\Psi(\text{o})|^2$ are in close agreement with the values obtained from E.S.R. experiments (see Table 2.1 and Table 5.1).

The singlet-doublet and singlet-triplet splittings in silicon and germanium respectively are usually called 'valley-orbit' splittings and have been measured in E.S.R. experiments on strained crystals, as also has the deformation potential. The latter quantity is essentially a measure of the shift of energy bands with applied strain.

§1.4

SHALLOW ACCEPTOR STATES IN SILICON AND GERMANIUM

Group III atoms, such as boron, aluminium, gallium, and indium, can be introduced into silicon and germanium as substitutional impurities. One of the covalent bonds at a lattice site occupied by a Group III atom is not completed and, at low temperatures, the 'hole' is bound to the impurity centre. At higher temperatures an electron can be taken from a host atom bond to complete the bonding at the Group III atom, and a hole is released into the valence band. The ionization energies of these shallow acceptor centres are $\sim$0·05 eV. Because of the degeneracy of the valence band at the zone centre, the theory of shallow acceptor centres is more complicated than for shallow donor centres.

In the 'tightly-bound' electron approximation, crystal wave functions (wave functions which describe an electron in the crystal as a whole) are constructed from atomic wave functions. For silicon and germanium the valence-band wave functions are constructed by sp^3 hybridization of atomic wave functions. Thus, at the zone centre, the valence band would be six-fold degenerate (including spin) in the absence of spin-orbit coupling. The effect of spin-orbit coupling is to lift partially this degeneracy, giving a four-fold degenerate band corresponding to atomic $J = \frac{3}{2}$ states, and a lower two-fold degenerate state corresponding to atomic $J = \frac{1}{2}$ states.

According to Kohn[11] the total wave function of an acceptor state can be written in the form

$$\Psi(\mathbf{r}) = \sum_{j=1}^{6} F_j(\mathbf{r})\psi_j(\mathbf{r}) \qquad (1.21)$$

where $F_j(\mathbf{r})$ is again an envelope function and the $\psi_j(\mathbf{r})$ are valence-band functions which have p-character near a lattice site.

§1.5
DEEP-LYING IMPURITY STATES IN SILICON AND GERMANIUM

In addition to the Group III and Group V impurity atoms, many other elements introduce energy levels between the valence and conduction bands. Apart from lithium, these energy levels lie much deeper in the band gap than the shallow impurity states introduced by Group III and Group V atoms (see Fig. 1.4).

These impurity atoms may, in general, enter the host lattice either substitutionally or interstitially and may or may not be electrically active.[15] The transition metals are an important class of elements which introduce electrically active impurities into silicon and germanium. Because of their low solubilities ($10^{14} - 10^{17} \text{cm}^{-3}$) the E.S.R. technique is an important tool for studying their properties. The charge states of these impurities can be altered by varying the position of the Fermi level in the energy gap. This can be accomplished by diffusing the impurity into a host crystal of controlled shallow impurity content.

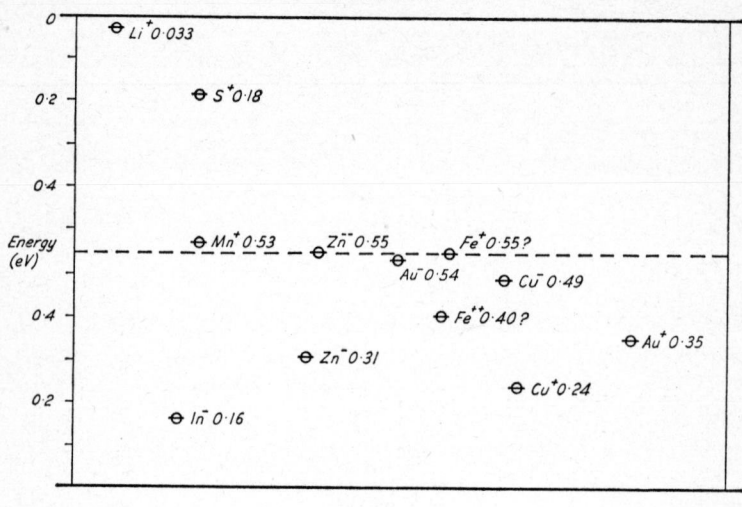

(a)

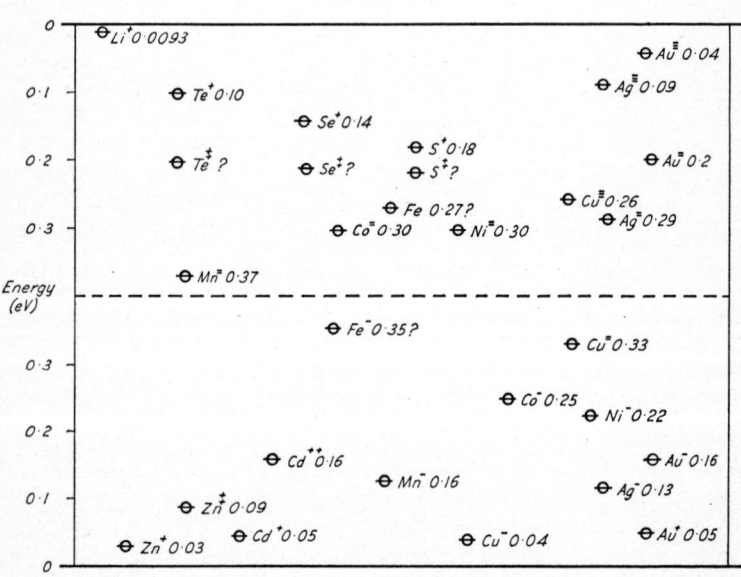

(b)

As these impurity states are deep-lying, the hydrogen-like effective mass theory does not apply. The E.S.R. technique has helped towards an improved understanding of the charge state of the impurities, of their position in relation to the host lattice, and of their solubilities.

§1.6

THE ENERGY-BAND STRUCTURE IN GROUP III–V COMPOUNDS

The energy-band structures of the Group III–V compounds are similar in many respects to those of the Group IV semiconductors, although the details of the structures have not been elucidated to as great an extent as they have for silicon and germanium.[2]

The valence-band maxima are predicted to occur very close to, but not at, the centre of the zone, to be two-fold degenerate (not including spin), and to have a third-band split-off by spin-orbit coupling. The conduction-band minima are predicted to lie on the $\langle 100 \rangle$ or $\langle 111 \rangle$ directions in reciprocal space or at the zone centre.

From many experimental points of view, only a knowledge of the band 'edges' is necessary. However, cyclotron resonance experiments at microwave frequencies, which directly yield electron and hole effective masses at the band edges, have not been very fruitful, except for InSb, since crystals of a high enough degree of purity have not been available.

Experiments which indirectly yield information about the energy-band structure (e.g. optical absorption, magneto-resistance) appear to confirm the above picture of the band edges.

Fig. 1.4. Deep-lying impurity states in (*a*) silicon and (*b*) germanium. The ionization energies are measured from the conduction-band and valence-band edges in the upper and lower halves of the figure respectively.

Lithium is included since, although it is not a Group IV substitutional donor impurity, its ionization energy is of the same order of magnitude. (After N. B. Hannay;[15] by courtesy of the Reinhold Publishing Corporation.)

§1.7

IMPURITY STATES IN GROUP III–V COMPOUNDS

The evidence suggests that Group II impurity atoms enter the crystal lattice substitutionally, replacing the Group III host atoms, and that Group VI impurity atoms replace Group V host atoms, forming acceptor and donor centres respectively. Group IV atoms can also enter the host lattice substitutionally, tending to replace the larger of the two host atoms.[2]

Group III–V compounds have not yet been prepared to the same degree of purity as silicon and germanium, and the effect of residual impurities introduced during the crystal-growing process is often very important (concentration of residual impurities $> 10^{14}$ cm^{-3}).

A simple hydrogen-like model predicts an impurity ionization energy

$$E_I = \frac{m^* e^4}{2\epsilon^2 \hbar^2} \tag{1.22}$$

which should be a fairly good approximation for materials with large dielectric constants and charge carriers of small effective mass. For indium arsenide this model predicts $E_I = -0 \cdot 002$ eV for donors and $\sim 0 \cdot 05$ eV for acceptors. The corresponding radii of the 'is-like' orbits are 310 Å and ~ 12 Å respectively. Other Group III–V compounds have donor impurity ionization energies, predicted by this model, in the range $-0 \cdot 0007$ eV to $-0 \cdot 008$ eV.

As a consequence of these very large donor 'radii', there is considerable interaction between neighbouring impurities, and the impurity energy levels merge into an 'impurity band'. Hence it is difficult to study the properties of isolated donor impurities because of the relatively low degree of purity of the available materials.

References

1. See, for instance, Kittel, C., *Introduction to Solid State Physics*, 2nd ed., Chapter 12 (John Wiley & Sons Inc., 1960), and Dekker, A. J., *Solid State Physics*, Chapter 10 (Macmillan & Co. Ltd, 1958).
2. Hilsum, C., and Rose-Innes, A. C., *Semiconducting III-V Compounds*, p. 5 (Pergamon Press, 1961).
3. Inokuchi, H., and Akamatu, H., *Solid State Physics*, Vol. 12 (Academic Press Inc., 1961).

4. Ingram, D. J. E., *Free Radicals as studied by Electron Spin Resonance* (Butterworths, 1958).
5. England, T. S., and Schneider, E. E., *Physica*, 1951, **17**, 221.
6. Portis, A. M., Kip, A. F., Kittel, C., and Brattain, W. H., *Phys. Rev.*, 1953, **90**, 988.
7. Fletcher, R. C., Yager, W. A., Pearson, G. L., Holden, A. N., Read, W. T., and Merritt, F. R., *Phys. Rev.*, 1954, **94**, 1392.
8. Wannier, G., *Phys. Rev.*, 1937, **52**, 191.
9. Kleinman, L., and Phillips, J. C., *Phys. Rev.*, 1960, **118**, 1153.
10. Phillips, J. C., *Phys. Rev.*, 1958, **112**, 685.
11. Kohn, W., *Solid State Physics*, Vol. 5, p. 257 (Academic Press Inc., 1957).
12. Wilson, D. K., and Feher, G., *Phys. Rev.*, 1961, **124**, 1068.
13. Wilson, D. K., *Phys. Rev.*, 1964, **134**, A265.
14. Kopferman, H., *Nuclear Moments*, p. 118 (Academic Press, 1958).
15. Hannay, N. B., (Ed.), *Semiconductors*, Chapter 8 (Reinhold Publishing Corporation, 1959).

Chapter 2

Group V Impurities in Silicon

§2.1

HYPERFINE INTERACTIONS AND THE DONOR-ELECTRON
WAVE FUNCTION FOR SHALLOW IMPURITY STATES

Shortly after the work of Portis et al.,[1] Fletcher et al.[2] observed
E.S.R. spectra in phosphorus-, arsenic-, and antimony-doped
silicon ($N_d \sim 10^{17}$ cm^{-3}) at 4·2°K. The spectra were identified
with neutral phosphorus, arsenic, and antimony centres by
the characteristic hyperfine splitting into $(2I+1)$ lines.

These experimental results can be described by a spin Hamiltonian of the simple form

$$\mathcal{H} = g\beta \mathbf{S}.\mathbf{H} + a\mathbf{S}.\mathbf{I} \qquad (2.1)$$

where a is given by the Fermi-Segrè expression for the electron-
donor nucleus 'contact' hyperfine interaction. Because of the cubic
symmetry of the electron wave function, the magnetic dipole-
dipole hyperfine interaction term averages to zero.

From equation (2.1) we obtain

$$E(m_s, m_I) = g\beta H m_s + a m_s m_I \qquad (2.2)$$

where m_s and m_I are the electron spin and nuclear magnetic
quantum numbers respectively, and resonance is observed at
frequencies given by

$$\hbar\omega = g\beta H + a m_I \qquad (2.3)$$

Since m_I can range from $-I$ to $+I$ in integral steps, there are
$(2I+1)$ lines with separation equal to a.

The spectra in phosphorus- and arsenic-doped silicon consist
of two and four lines respectively (nuclear spin $I = \frac{1}{2}$ for P^{31} and
$\frac{3}{2}$ for As^{75}). In the antimony-doped sample there are two over-
lapping spectra consisting of six and eight lines. The number,

relative intensity, and relative separation between the lines are consistent with hyperfine interactions between the donor electrons and Sb^{121} ($I = \frac{5}{2}$) and Sb^{123} ($I = \frac{7}{2}$) impurity nuclei. The values for $|\Psi'(o)|^2$ calculated from these observed hyperfine splittings are shown in Table 2.1.

For phosphorus-doped silicon Kohn[3] calculated $|\Psi'(o)|^2$ on the basis of the corrected effective mass theory and obtained $|\Psi'(o)|^2 = 0.41 \times 10^{24}$ cm^{-3} in close agreement with the experimental result.

Fletcher *et al.*[4] investigated the saturation behaviour of the hyperfine lines and concluded that they were 'inhomogeneously' broadened. The source of this broadening lies in the hyperfine interaction between the donor electron and the 4.7 per cent abundant Si^{29} nuclei ($I = \frac{1}{2}$) within its orbit (the Si^{28} nucleus has zero magnetic moment).

If this interaction is included in the spin Hamiltonian, then we have

$$\mathcal{H} = g\beta \mathbf{S} \cdot \mathbf{H} + a\mathbf{S} \cdot \mathbf{I} + \sum_L a' \mathbf{S} \cdot \mathbf{I}' \qquad (2.4)$$

Here

$$a' = \frac{8\pi}{3} g g_N' \beta \beta_N |\Psi(\mathbf{r}_L)|^2 \qquad (2.5)$$

where $\mathbf{I}'$ and g_N' are the nuclear spin and g-factor respectively of the Si^{29} nuclei, and the summation is over all the lattice sites occupied by Si^{29} nuclei.

The shift in the magnetic field experienced by a particular donor electron will be

$$\Delta H = \frac{8\pi}{3} g_N' \beta_N \sum_L |\Psi(\mathbf{r}_L)|^2 m_L' \qquad (2.6)$$

where m_L' is the magnetic quantum number of the Si^{29} nucleus at the Lth lattice site. The results of the summation differ from donor atom to donor atom. Kohn[3] assumed that $\mathbf{r}_L$ and m_L' varied randomly and obtained

$$\Delta H_{r.m.s.} = \overline{(\Delta H^2)}^{1/2} = f^{1/2} \left(\frac{8\pi}{3} g_N' \beta_N \right) \left(\sum_L' \left| \Psi(\mathbf{r}_L) \right|^4 \right)^{1/2} \qquad (2.7)$$

where f is the natural fractional abundance of Si^{29} nuclei, and the sum runs over all lattice sites with the exception of that occupied by the donor nucleus.

Kohn fitted this result to the observed line width by varying the parameter k_0 [see equation (1.9)] and found $k_0/k_{max} = 0.7$ to an estimated accuracy of within 25 per cent.

In the electron nuclear double resonance (E.N.D.O.R.) technique developed by Feher[5] both a microwave and a radio-frequency magnetic field are applied to the sample. The large magnetic field H is set to one of the donor hyperfine lines [equation (2.3)] and the electron resonance absorption is saturated, resulting in a reduction of the signal. The frequency of the radio-frequency field is swept through the nuclear transition frequencies ($\Delta m_I = \pm 1, \Delta m_L' = \pm 1$), thereby changing the populations of the electronic levels and desaturating the line. This leads to a change in the level of the electron resonance signal which can be recorded.

The reason for the higher resolving power of this technique can be seen by considering the donor-nucleus transitions. These are specified by $\Delta m_s = \Delta m_L' = 0$ and $\Delta m_I = \pm 1$; the $\Delta m_s \Delta m_L'$ terms arising from the last term in equation (2.4) do not broaden the line. The reduction in width of these transitions is about three orders of magnitude, from 10 Mc/s to 10 kc/s.

Studying the Si^{29} transitions in arsenic-doped silicon[5] ($N_d = 8 \times 10^{16}$ cm^{-3}) yields information about the amplitude of the donor-electron wave function at the sites within its orbit occupied by Si^{29} nuclei. Unfortunately $|\Psi(\mathbf{r}_L)|^2$ does not decrease monotonically with increasing $\mathbf{r}_L$, owing to interference between the six factors $\exp[i(\mathbf{k}_{0j}.\mathbf{r})]$ in the donor wave function. Hence a knowledge of the frequencies of the Si^{29} transitions in the E.N.D.O.R. spectrum is not alone sufficient to identify the lattice sites. Two additional pieces of information, available from the E.N.D.O.R. spectrum, assist in identifying the lines. Firstly, the relative amplitudes of the lines has to be consistent with the number of equivalent occupied lattice sites. Secondly, from the angular variation of the additional anisotropic fine structure on the lines, the symmetry of a particular lattice point with respect to the donor-impurity centre is determined.

The experimental values for a', the isotropic part of the hyperfine interaction, agreed to within 50 per cent with the theory of

Kohn and Luttinger, but there is no satisfactory theory for the anisotropic part as yet.

By using material enriched in Si^{28} nuclei (isotopic purity 99·88 per cent of Si^{28} nuclei), Feher[6] was able to reduce the line width in a phosphorus-doped sample by about an order of magnitude to 0·22 gauss. These extremely narrow lines enabled the material to be used as the basis of a two-level maser (see §6.6).

§2.2

g-VALUES OF DONOR ELECTRONS

The measured g-values are isotropic for all Group V donors and their magnitudes are shown in Table 2.1. It will be noticed that $(g-g_e)$ is small ($\sim 10^{-3}$) in all cases.

Roth[7] calculated the g-factors of conduction electrons in silicon and germanium on the basis of a 'two-band' model, i.e. only the momentum matrix elements between the conduction band and the valence band were considered. The expressions obtained, for an electron confined to a single valley, were:

$$g_\parallel - g_e = -\left(\frac{\delta'}{\Delta E}\right)\left(\frac{m_e}{m_\perp} - 1\right) \qquad (2.8)$$

and

$$g_\perp - g_e = \left(\frac{\delta'}{\Delta E}\right)\left(\frac{m_e}{m_\parallel} - 1\right) \qquad (2.9)$$

Here δ' is two-thirds of the spin-orbit splitting of the valence band at $k = 0$, ΔE is the energy difference between the conduction-band and valence-band edges and $m_\parallel$, $m_\perp$ are respectively the longitudinal and transverse effective masses for a single valley.

The reason for the close relation between the expressions for the electron effective mass and its g-value is that inter-band momentum matrix elements occur in both cases.

In general, the electron spin magnetic moment μ and the effective spin vector operator $\mathbf{S}$ are related by an expression of the form

$$\mu = \beta \mathbf{g}.\mathbf{S} \qquad (2.10)$$

where $\mathbf{g}$ is a symmetric second-rank tensor.

For an electron in the jth valley

$$g^j = \begin{pmatrix} g_\perp & 0 & 0 \\ 0 & g_\perp & 0 \\ 0 & 0 & g_\| \end{pmatrix} \qquad (2.11)$$

where the principal axes of this tensor coincide with those of the tensor for the effective mass.

In an E.S.R. experiment, the measured interaction energy $\beta\mathbf{H}.\mathbf{g}.\mathbf{S}$ is an average over the six equivalent valleys, taking into account their relative populations.

The relation (2.11) for g^j can be written[8]

$$g^j = g_\perp \begin{pmatrix} 1 & 0 & 0 \\ 0 & 1 & 0 \\ 0 & 0 & 1 \end{pmatrix} + (g_\| - g_\perp)\begin{pmatrix} 0 & 0 & 0 \\ 0 & 0 & 0 \\ 0 & 0 & 1 \end{pmatrix} \qquad (2.12)$$

$$= g_\perp \mathbf{1} + (g_\| - g_\perp)\mathbf{U}^j \qquad (2.13)$$

and

$$\langle \beta\mathbf{H}.\mathbf{g}.\mathbf{S} \rangle_{\mathrm{AV}} = \beta\mathbf{H}.\left\{ \sum_{j=1}^{6} (\alpha_j)^2 [g_\perp \mathbf{1} + (g_\| - g_\perp)\mathbf{U}^j] \right\}.\mathbf{S} \qquad (2.14)$$

where the α^j are given in equation (1.16).

For the singlet ground state all the α_j are equal and

$$\langle \beta\mathbf{H}.\mathbf{g}.\mathbf{S} \rangle_{\mathrm{AV}} = \beta\mathbf{H}.[g_\perp + \tfrac{2}{6}(g_\| - g_\perp)]\mathbf{1}.\mathbf{S}$$

$$= (\tfrac{2}{3}g_\perp + \tfrac{1}{3}g_\|)\beta\mathbf{H}.\mathbf{S}$$

$$= g_0\beta\mathbf{H}.\mathbf{S} \qquad (2.15)$$

Thus the measured g-value should be isotropic, as is indeed observed.

In silicon

$$\delta = 0.04 \text{ eV}$$

$$\Delta E = 4 \text{ eV}$$

$$m_e/m_\perp = 5.3$$

$$m_e/m_\| = 1.02$$

TABLE 2.1 Parameters of donor-impurity atoms in silicon at $1\cdot25°$K*

Donor impurity	Ionization energy (eV)	$g-g_{C.E.}$† $(\times 10^4)$	Nuclear spin I	a (Mc/s)	$|\Psi(o)|^2$ $(\times 10^{-24}\ \mathrm{cm}^{-3})$ Experiment	Theory	Width of hyperfine components (gauss)
Sb[121]	0·043	−1·7±1	$\frac{5}{2}$	186·802±0·005	1·18		2·3
Sb[123]	0·043		$\frac{7}{2}$	101·516±0·004	1·18		
P[31]	0·045	−2·5±1	$\frac{1}{2}$	117·53 ±0·02	0·43	0·4	2·5
As[75]	0·054	−3·8±1	$\frac{3}{2}$	198·366±0·02	1·73		2·9
As[76]	0·054		2	198·35 ±0·02	1·73		
Bi[209]	0·071	+15±1	$\frac{9}{2}$	1475·5 ±0·1	14		4·5

* These figures were taken from Feher[5] apart from the ionization energies, which were taken from Kohn.[9]

† $g_{C.E.}$ (conduction electrons) $= 1\cdot99875 + 0\cdot00010$.
g_e (free electrons) $= 2\cdot00229 \pm 0\cdot000026$.

TABLE 2.2 Experimental and calculated values for $\delta g_{\parallel}$ and $\delta g_{\perp}$ in silicon*

Donor impurity	g_0	$g_{\parallel}-g_{\perp}$	$\delta g_{\parallel}$ Experiment	Calculation	$\delta g_{\perp}$ Experiment	Calculation
Sb	1·99858±0·0001	$(1\cdot13\pm0\cdot05)\times10^{-3}$	−0·0030	−0·0027	−0·0041	−0·0036
P	1·98850±0·0001	$(1\cdot04\pm0\cdot04)\times10^{-3}$	−0·0131		−0·0141	
As	1·99837±0·0001	$(1\cdot10\pm0\cdot05)\times10^{-3}$	−0·0032		−0·0043	

* The experimental values are taken from Wilson and Feher[10] and the calculated values from Liu.[11]

and from equations (2.8) and (2.9)

$$g_{\parallel} - g_0 = \delta g_{\parallel} = -0 \cdot 028$$

$$g_{\perp} - g_0 = \delta g_{\perp} \simeq -0 \cdot 005$$

and

$$g_0 - g_e \simeq -0 \cdot 013 \tag{2.16}$$

Note that in this model $\delta g_{\perp}$ is negligible compared with $\delta g_{\parallel}$, whereas measurements on phosphorus-doped silicon[10] have indicated that $|\delta g_{\perp}| > |\delta g_{\parallel}|$ (see Table 2.2). Liu[11] has calculated the g-values of conduction electrons in silicon using crystal wave functions and finds that the dominant contribution to δg comes from the deep-lying 2p state, because of its large spin-orbit splitting. Liu found $\delta g_{\parallel} = -0 \cdot 0027$ and $\delta g_{\perp} = -0 \cdot 0036$ in good agreement with the experimental results for antimony centres (see Table 2.2), which are the 'shallowest' of the donor centres. The value for δg_0 calculated from Liu's results for $\delta g_{\parallel}$ and $\delta g_{\perp}$ is $-0 \cdot 0033$, which is also in good agreement with the experimental results (see Table 2.2).

It can be seen from Table 2.1 that the g-shifts for the donor centres increase with increasing donor ionization energy except for bismuth. Although bismuth is a Group V impurity, it has a considerably larger ionization energy than the other donor centres. Hence the theoretical treatment of Kohn and Luttinger[12] is not expected to apply to bismuth.

Spin-orbit coupling to the donor atom appears to make very little contribution to the g-shift, since δg varies by a factor of only a little over 2 from antimony to arsenic, whereas the atomic spin-orbit coupling constants differ by more than an order of magnitude.

§2.3

HYPERFINE INTERACTION AND g-VALUES IN STRAINED CRYSTALS

The E.S.R. experiments so far described have yielded information only about the ground states of the various donor centres. The nearest excited states to the ground state are, as we have seen, the approximately degenerate set of doublet and triplet states, which are split off from the ground state by the 'valley-orbit' interaction. Since optical transitions between the ground state and the doublet/triplet level are forbidden, the valley-orbit splitting cannot be obtained directly from the infra-red absorption spectra of the donor centres.

When there is uniaxial stress, the equivalence of the six conduction-band minima (valleys) is destroyed, and admixture of the first excited state and the singlet ground state occurs.

If the energy shift of the jth valley is $S\epsilon_j$, which is due to a strain S, where the ϵ_j are proportional to the deformation potential D_u, and $\psi_s^{(1)}$ is the wave function for the ground state after admixture, then, for small strains, perturbation theory yields[3]

$$\psi_s^{(1)} = \psi^{(1)} + S \sum_{i=2}^{6} \frac{1}{E^{(1)} - E^{(i)}} \left(\sum_{j=1}^{6} \alpha_j^{(1)} \epsilon_j \, \alpha_j^{(1)} \right) \psi^{(i)} \quad (2.17)$$

This can be written more generally as

$$\psi_s^{(1)} = C_1 \psi^{(1)} + S \sum_{i=2}^{6} C_i \psi^{(i)} \quad (2.18)$$

and normalization requires

$$1 = C_1^2 + S^2 \sum_{i=2}^{6} C_i^2 \quad (2.19)$$

To interpret the observed strain-dependence of the hyperfine splitting in the E.S.R. spectra of the donor centres, an expression for $|\psi_s^{(1)}(0)|^2$ is required.

Remembering that the $\psi^{(i)}$ ($i \neq 1$) have nodes at the donor nucleus, equation (2.18) yields

$$|\psi_s^{(1)}(0)|^2 = C_1^2 |\psi^1(0)|^2$$

or

$$\frac{|\psi_s^{(1)}(0)|^2}{|\psi^1(0)|^2} = 1 - S^2 \sum_{i=2}^{6} C_i^2 \quad (2.20)$$

i.e., the first-order effect of the strain on the hyperfine splitting vanishes. Nevertheless the second-order effect yields 5 per cent changes in the observed hyperfine splitting for experimentally attainable strains.

The g-values of the donor electrons are also affected by strains, for two reasons. Firstly, the populations of the six valleys will no longer be the same since their equivalence has been destroyed. Hence, an average over the populations of the valleys results in an anisotropic g-value. Secondly, the g-value of an electron moving in one valley will change with applied stress, since the momentum matrix elements with nearby bands are strain-dependent.

The spin-lattice relaxation time of the donor electrons is also affected by strains. This effect will be discussed when we consider relaxation mechanisms (see pp. 38 to 43).

Hyperfine interaction

Wilson and Feher[10] have shown that a uniaxial stress in the [100] direction causes admixture of the wave functions for the singlet ground state and for one component only of the doublet/triplet excited state. Hence,

$$\frac{(h.f.s.)_{\text{strain}}}{(h.f.s.)_0} = \frac{1}{2}\left[1 + \left(1 + \frac{x}{6}\right)\left(1 + \frac{x}{3} + \frac{x^2}{4}\right)^{-1/2}\right] \quad (2.21)$$

where

$$x = \frac{D_u S'}{E_{12}} \quad (2.22)$$

Here E_{12} is the valley-orbit splitting and S' is given by

$$T/S' = \tfrac{1}{2}(C_{11} - C_{12})$$

where T is the applied stress in the [100] direction and $\tfrac{1}{2}(C_{11} - C_{12})$ is the appropriate elastic constant.[13]

Equation (2.21) reduces to the quadratic form

$$\frac{(h.f.s.)_{\text{strain}}}{(h.f.s.)_0} = 1 - \frac{x^2}{18} \quad (2.23)$$

for small strains.

The observed reduction in hyperfine splitting with applied strain in phosphorus-doped silicon is shown in Fig. 2.1.

Equation (2.21) was fitted to the experimental results by putting $E_{12}/D_u = 1\cdot 32 \times 10^{-3}$. Fig. 2.2 shows the result of plotting the values of x calculated from equation (2.21), using the experimentally observed values of $(h.f.s.)_{\text{strain}}/(h.f.s.)_0$, versus the actual strain, deduced from the applied stress and the known elastic

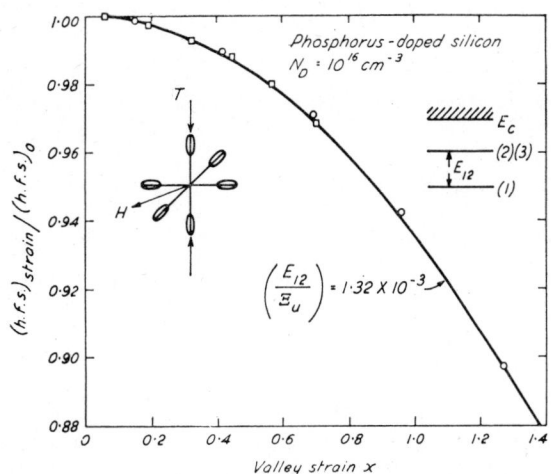

Fig. 2.1. Reduction of hyperfine splitting in phosphorus-doped silicon at $1\cdot25°$K, owing to uniaxial compression in a [100] direction. The curve was fitted to the experimental points by assuming $E_{12}/D_u = 1\cdot 32 \times 10^3$. (After Wilson and Feher.[10])

constants of silicon. The validity of equation (2.21) is affirmed by the linearity of the lines in Fig. 2.2, and the values for E_{12}/D_u, obtained from the slopes of the lines, are shown in Table 2.3.

To determine the valley-orbit splittings, the deformation potential D_u must be known. Optical absorption experiments have indicated that the energies of higher excited states, whose wave functions have nodes at the donor-impurity nucleus, are independent of the donor species. By assuming that the energy of the doublet/triplet state is also independent of the donor species, and using the observed donor ionization energies, an average value for D_u can be calculated.

3

If E' is the energy of the doublet/triplet state and E_I is the donor ionization energy, then

$$E' - E_I = \left(\frac{E_{12}}{D_u}\right)D_u \qquad (2.24)$$

or

$$E_I + \left(\frac{E_{12}}{D_u}\right)D_u = \text{constant} \qquad (2.25)$$

for antimony, phosphorus, and arsenic centres. Using the measured values[10] of E_{12}/D_u, the average value obtained for D_u is 11 ± 1 eV.

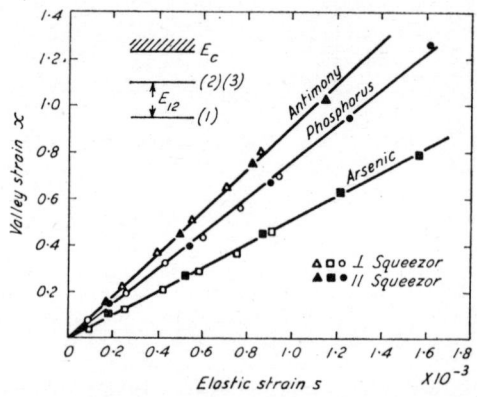

FIG. 2.2. Compression in a [100] direction causes the elastic strain s for donor impurities in silicon at $1 \cdot 25°$K. The continuous lines correspond to the values of E_{12}/D_u listed in Table 2.3. (After Wilson and Feher.[10])

The doublet/triplet state corresponds in energy to the six-fold degenerate ground state in the effective mass approximation and this energy is calculated to be -29×10^{-3} eV. Using the above value for D_u in equation (2.24), the value obtained for E' is $-30 \cdot 0 \times 10^{-3}$ eV, which is in good agreement with the theoretical value.

g-values

The g-value in a strained crystal is given by an expression of the form of equation (2.14) when only the valley-repopulation effect is taken into account.

The two admixed states resulting from a [100] compressive stress are represented by[10]

$$\alpha^j_{\text{strain}} = (\alpha_A, \ \alpha_A, \ \alpha_B, \ \alpha_B, \ \alpha_B, \ \alpha_B) \tag{2.26}$$

where

$$\alpha_A{}^2 = \frac{1}{4}\left[1 \mp \left(x+\frac{2}{3}\right)\left(x^2+\frac{4x}{3}+4\right)^{-1/2}\right] \tag{2.27}$$

$$\alpha_B{}^2 = \frac{1}{8}\left[1 \pm \left(x+\frac{2}{3}\right)\left(x^2+\frac{4x}{3}+4\right)^{-1/2}\right] \tag{2.28}$$

and the upper and lower signs refer to the lower and higher of the two admixed states respectively.

Hence

$$\langle\beta\mathbf{H}.\mathbf{g}.\mathbf{S}\rangle_{\text{Av}} = \beta\mathbf{H}.\left[(2\alpha_A{}^2+4\alpha_B{}^2)g_\perp \mathbf{1}\right]$$

$$+2(g_\parallel-g_\perp)\alpha_A{}^2\begin{pmatrix} 0 & & \\ & 0 & \\ & & 1 \end{pmatrix}$$

$$+2(g_\parallel-g_\perp)\alpha_B{}^2\begin{pmatrix} 0 & & \\ & 1 & \\ & & 0 \end{pmatrix}$$

$$+2(g_\parallel-g_\perp)\alpha_B{}^2\begin{pmatrix} 1 & & \\ & 0 & \\ & & 0 \end{pmatrix} \tag{2.29}$$

Remembering that normalization requires $2\alpha_A{}^2+4\alpha_B{}^2 = 1$, this leads to

$$\langle\beta\mathbf{H}.\mathbf{g}.\mathbf{S}\rangle_{\text{Av}}=$$

$$\beta\mathbf{H}.\begin{vmatrix} g_\perp+2(g_\parallel-g_\perp)\alpha_B{}^2 & 0 & 0 \\ 0 & g_\perp+2(g_\parallel-g_\perp)\alpha_B{}^2 & 0 \\ 0 & 0 & g_\perp+2(g_\parallel-g_\perp)\alpha_A{}^2 \end{vmatrix}.\mathbf{S}$$

which can be written in the form

$$\langle \beta \mathbf{H}.\mathbf{g}.\mathbf{S} \rangle_{Av} = \beta \mathbf{H}. \begin{vmatrix} g_\perp' & & \\ & g_\perp' & \\ & & g_\parallel' \end{vmatrix} .\mathbf{S} \qquad (2.30)$$

For a **g**-tensor of this form, the observed g-value is given by

$$g^2 = (g_\parallel')^2 \cos^2\theta + (g_\perp')^2 \sin^2\theta \qquad (2.31)$$

where θ is the angle between the applied magnetic field and the [100] axis. By using the explicit expressions for $g_\parallel'$, $g_\perp'$, α_A^2, α_B^2, by making use of $g_0 = \frac{1}{3}g_\parallel + \frac{2}{3}g_\perp$, and remembering that $(g_\parallel - g_\perp)/g_\perp$ is small, we find

$$g - g_0 = \frac{1}{6}(g_\parallel - g_\perp)(1 - \frac{3}{2}\sin^2\theta)\left[1 - (3x+2)\left(x^2 + \frac{4x}{3} + 4\right)^{-1/2}\right] \qquad (2.32)$$

Then, for large applied stresses $(-x \gg 1)$, and for **H** in the [100] direction (i.e., parallel to the valley axis)

$$g = g_\parallel \qquad (2.33)$$

If **H** is perpendicular to the stress, then

$$g = g_\perp \qquad (2.34)$$

These results are consistent with the notion of the electron spending its time in two opposite valleys only.

From experiments made with the applied stress along the [100] direction, and with $\theta = 90°$, Wilson and Feher[10] obtained $g_\parallel - g_\perp \simeq 10^{-3}$ by fitting expression (2.32) to the experimental results (see Table 2.2). They also concluded that $g_\perp < g_\parallel$, since the g-factor decreased with increasing strain.

By making measurements with **H** in the (110) plane, and with x as a variable parameter, it was confirmed that $(g - g_0)$ vanished when **H** was in the [111] direction, as predicted by equation (2.32) (see Fig. 2.3). The value obtained for $(g_\parallel - g_\perp)$ using this method agreed with those obtained by the first method.

The shift in the one-valley g-factor is due to strain-dependent momentum matrix elements between a valley and nearby energy

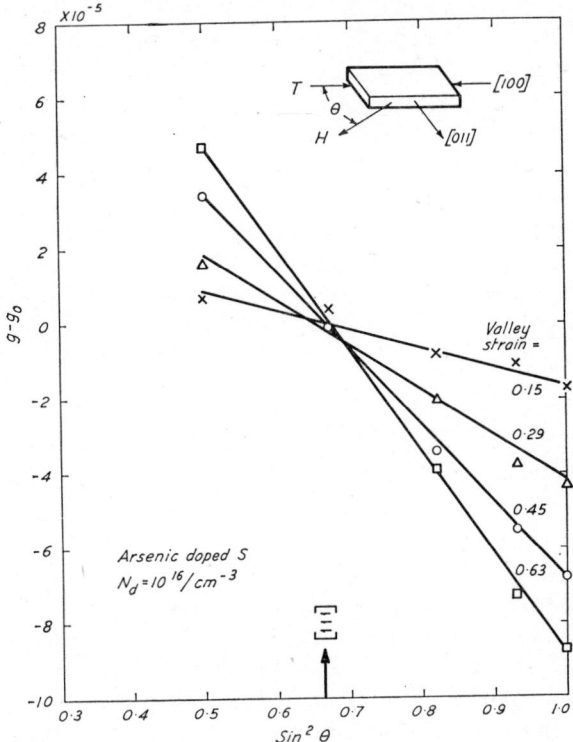

FIG. 2.3. *g*-shift versus $\sin^2\theta$ in arsenic-doped silicon at $1\cdot25^\circ$K, where θ is the angle between the stress axis and the magnetic field for a uniaxial compression in the [100] direction. (After Wilson and Feher.[10])

bands. The resultant *g*-shift is given by[14]

$$g - g_0 = \frac{A}{3}\left(\frac{T}{C_{44}}\right)\left(1 - \tfrac{3}{2}\sin^2\theta\right) \qquad (2.35)$$

where A is a constant and T is an applied stress in the [111] direction. **H** is applied in the (110) plane and θ is the angle between **H** and the direction of the applied stress. The one-valley *g*-shift was also measured by Wilson and Feher[10] who found that it vanished for T in the [100] direction, in accordance with equation (2.35).

It is this fact, and that the 'valley-repopulation' effect vanishes for stresses in the [111] direction, which allow the two effects contributing to g-shifts in strained crystals to be studied independently if suitable stress axes are chosen.

By comparing the experimental results for the one-valley g-shift with equation (2.35), Wilson and Feher[10] obtained for A the value 0.44 ± 0.04.

Thus it may be deduced that the nearest band, which is admixed with a conduction-band valley [$\Delta_{2'}$, see Fig. 1.2(a)], is separated from the donor ground state by an energy much greater than E_{12}.

§2.4

NON-LOCALIZED ELECTRONS

In the first observation of E.S.R. in silicon,[1] a single resonance line was observed in a powdered sample of n-type material ($N_d \simeq 2 \times 10^{18}$ cm^{-3}; $\rho = 0.01$ to 0.02 ohm cm at $300°$K) over the temperature range $300°$K to $4.2°$K. The susceptibility χ'' was proportional to T^{-1} above about $50°$K and below this temperature was independent of temperature. This was interpreted as indicating that the degeneracy temperature of the assembly of electrons was about $30°$K. Hence it was deduced that the resonance line was due to conduction electrons. The shape of the line was 'Lorentzian' (homogeneously broadened), indicating that the width of the line was due to a lifetime effect, and the line width increased from about 2 gauss at $4.4°$K to about 30 gauss at $300°$K.

Except in samples of medium donor-impurity concentration, and at low temperatures, the spin resonance of non-localized electrons cannot be observed in single-crystal specimens, for two reasons. Firstly, the energy losses due to eddy currents at the microwave frequency damp the cavity Q-factor prohibitively. Secondly, only those electrons moving within the skin depth can contribute to the resonance signal.

The skin depth d is given by

$$d = \sqrt{\left(\frac{\rho}{\pi\mu_0\nu}\right)} \qquad (2.36)$$

where ρ is the resistivity of the material and ν is the frequency of the microwaves. For $\rho = 0\cdot01$ ohm cm and $\nu = 10$ Gc/s, $d = 50$ microns.

If a powdered sample is used, with particle diameter $\ll d$, then both the above objections are overcome. The powder may be dispersed in paraffin wax to give a high-resistance sample,[1] but the intrinsic contact resistance between particles has been found to provide sufficient insulation.[15]

In powdered samples an additional resonance line is observed and is attributed to centres associated with the damaged surfaces of the particles.[5,15,16] At X-band frequencies this line can be a nuisance since it overlaps the conduction electron resonance line, but at Q-band frequencies the two lines are well resolved.

In those cases where single-crystal specimens may be used, the shape of the resonance line may be distorted, owing to the diffusion of the conduction electrons in and out of the skin depth. The electrons experience a microwave magnetic field of varying amplitude and phase, but Dyson[17] has found that the resonance line from a plate-like specimen of thickness t will be undistorted if $t \leqslant 4d$. For a silicon specimen of resistivity $0\cdot01$ ohm cm and with $\nu = 10$ Gc/s (X band), then $4d = 200$ microns, and for $\nu = 35$ Gc/s (Q band), $4d = 100$ microns.

In lightly doped specimens ($N_d \leqslant 5 \times 10^{17}$ cm^{-3} approximately) the number of electrons in the conduction band is given by

$$n_c = (2N_d)^{1/2}\left(\frac{2\pi m^* k T}{h^2}\right)^{3/4}\exp\left(-\frac{E_I}{2kT}\right) \qquad (2\cdot37)$$

and the conduction electron resonance cannot be observed until $T \geqslant 40°K$ approximately.

Electrons in an impurity band

Non-localized electrons may exist in either the true conduction band or in an impurity band. If the donor impurities are close enough together ($N_d \geqslant 10^{17}$ cm^{-3} approximately), such that their wave functions overlap to an appreciable extent, then an impurity band is said to be formed. The donor electrons may move from donor to donor and to this extent are de-localized, although their mobility is less than in the true conduction band.[18,19]

In samples of phosphorus-doped silicon with $N_d \geqslant 7 \times 10^{16}$ cm^{-3}

at liquid helium or hydrogen temperatures, 'satellite' lines are observed between the main hyperfine components. As the concentration of donor impurities is increased, these satellite lines grow in number and intensity, and, eventually, for N_d in the region of 10^{18} cm^{-3}, a single line only is observed at the position of the centre of gravity of the original hyperfine lines.

The satellite lines occurring mid-way between the main hyperfine lines are attributed to 'exchange-coupled' pairs of electrons from donor impurities lying particularly close together.[20]

For this situation the spin Hamiltonian is

$$\mathscr{H} = g\beta(S_{1_z}+S_{2_z})H_0 + A\mathbf{S}_1 . \mathbf{S}_2 + a(\mathbf{I}_1 . \mathbf{S}_1 + \mathbf{I}_2 . \mathbf{S}_2)$$
$$+ g_N\beta_N(I_{1_z}+I_{2_z})H_0 \tag{2.38}$$

where H_0 is in the z-direction.

Here $\mathbf{S}_1$, $\mathbf{S}_2$ are the two electron spins and $\mathbf{I}_1$, $\mathbf{I}_2$ the spins of the two phosphorus nuclei. $A\mathbf{S}_1 . \mathbf{S}_2$ is the exchange coupling between the two electrons of the interacting donor-impurity atoms.[21]

For $A \gg a$ the electrons are strongly coupled together and can be regarded as a system having total spin $\mathbf{S} = 1$, 0 and $M_s = 1, 0, -1$ and 0. So

$$E = g\beta H_0 M_s + \frac{A}{2}[S(S+1)-\tfrac{3}{2}] - \frac{a}{2}(M_s m_1 + M_s m_2)$$
$$+ g_N\beta_N H_0(m_1+m_2) \tag{2.39}$$

If the microwave magnetic field is given by $h_x \cos \omega t$, then the observed transitions are given by the selection rule $\Delta S = 0$, $\Delta M_s = \pm 1$ and

$$h\nu = g\beta H_0 + \frac{A}{2}[S(S+1)-\tfrac{3}{2}] + \frac{a}{2}(m_1+m_2) \tag{2.40}$$

In phosphorus-doped silicon there will be three satellite lines of spacing $a/2$ (as compared with a spacing a for the main hyperfine lines), and the intensities will be in the ratio 1 : 2 : 1. Of course the outer lines coincide with the main hyperfine components and are not observed.

Satellite lines attributed to clusters of more than two donor-impurity atoms have been observed.

The appearance of the satellite lines as N_d increases, and the eventual replacement of the hyperfine lines by a single line also marks the transition from a semiconductor to a metallic material $(N_d \sim 10^{19} \text{ cm}^{-3})$.

g-values of electrons in the conduction band

Feher[5] has measured the g-value of non-localized electrons in phosphorus-doped silicon $(N_d = 3 \times 10^{18} \text{ cm}^{-3})$ at X-band frequencies to a high degree of accuracy and found

$$g = 1 \cdot 99875 \pm 0 \cdot 00010$$

at $1 \cdot 25°\text{K}$. From measurements at $77°\text{K}$ on single-crystal specimens of phosphorus-doped silicon $(N_d \sim 10^{18} \text{ cm}^{-3})$ at Q-band frequencies, Lancaster, van Wyk and Schneider[22] found

$$g = 1 \cdot 9988 \pm 0 \cdot 0001$$

These measured g-values are, of course, an isotropic average over the six conduction-band minima.

The E.S.R. signal from an n-type silicon sample with $N_d \sim 10^{18} \text{ cm}^{-3}$ provides a very useful 'g-marker'. The sample is stable and exhibits a narrow, symmetric resonance line and is superior to other g-markers such as $CuSO_4$, D.P.P.H.,* or LiH in one or all of these respects. Gere[23] embedded n-type silicon of this impurity concentration, in powdered form, in polythene sheet, which could then be simply cut into samples of a convenient size.

Spin-lattice relaxation of conduction electrons

The observed conduction electron resonance lines are homogeneously broadened, the line width corresponding to a spin-lattice relaxation time of the order of 10^{-8} sec.

For such a lifetime broadened resonance line

$$\Delta\omega_{1/2} = 2T_2^{-1} \tag{2.41}$$

The relation between T_2 and T_1 has been investigated by Pines and Slichter.[24] If the frequency characteristic of the lattice vibrations (the reciprocal of the correlation time) is much less than the

* Diphenyl-picryl-hydrazyl

Larmor frequency, then Pines and Slichter, and Wangsness and Bloch[25] find $T_1 = T_2$ and

$$\Delta\omega_{1/2} = 2T_1^{-1} \qquad (2.42)$$

for an isotropic lattice structure, e.g. cubic crystals.

Thus

$$T_1^{-1} = \sqrt{3} \cdot (2\hbar)^{-1} g\beta\Delta H \qquad (2.43)$$

where ΔH is the line width between points of maximum slope of the first derivative of the absorption curve.

It is expected that the coupling between the spin and orbital magnetic moments of the electrons will be an important factor in the spin-lattice relaxation process, because of the large interaction between the orbital motion of the electron and the lattice.

Elliott[26] considered the effect of spin-orbit coupling on the magnetic resonance and found

$$\tau T_1^{-1} \sim (\delta g)^2 \qquad (2.44)$$

where τ is the relaxation time associated with the electrical resistivity of the material and δg is the difference between the free-electron g-factor and the observed g-factor.

Since $\tau \propto T^{-3/2}$ very nearly, equation (2.44) predicts $\Delta H \propto T^{3/2}$. Early work by Lancaster and Schneider[15] appeared to support this theory, although the proximity of the surface state resonance line made accurate line-width measurements difficult.

Yafet[14] has considered the modulation of the spin-orbit coupling by lattice vibrations as a time-dependent perturbation which can cause spin-lattice relaxation. For a conduction-band minimum not at $k = 0$, Yafet found

$$T_1^{-1} = \frac{2}{\pi^{3/2}\hbar} \cdot \frac{D^2}{\rho u^2} \cdot \left(\frac{2m^*kT}{\hbar^2}\right)^{5/2} \qquad (2.45)$$

where ρ is the density of silicon, u is the velocity of sound, and $D \sim D_u . a . \delta g$, where a is a length of the order of the lattice constant, or larger, and D_u is the deformation potential. Thus the line width is predicted to vary as $T^{5/2}$.

The results of further measurements by Lancaster *et al.*[22]

of the conduction electron resonance line width, at Q-band frequencies, are shown in Fig. 2.4.

From equation (2.45) the value obtained for T_1^{-1}, at 273°K, is $1·5 \times 10^7 \sec^{-1}$, using the following values for the parameters appearing in the equation: $D_u = 11·0$ eV, $a = 5·4$ Å, $\delta g = 3·5 \times 10^{-3}$, $\rho = 2·4 \times 10^3$ kg m^{-3}, $u = 5·4 \times 10^3$ msec^{-1}, $m^* = 0·35 \, m_e$ (density of states effective mass). Thus from equation

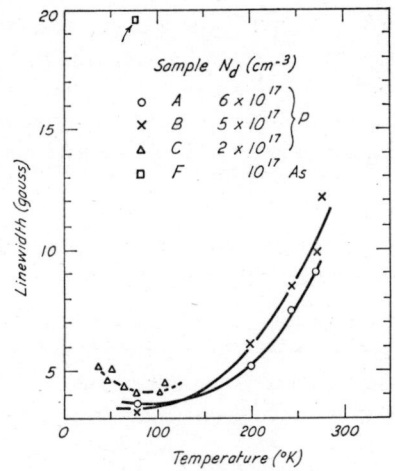

FIG. 2.4. Conduction electron resonance line width,* as measured at Q-band frequencies, versus temperature.

* Measured between points of maximum slope of the first derivative of the absorption curve.

(2.43) $\Delta H \gtrsim 1$ gauss, which agrees in order of magnitude with the experimental results.

Further, from equation (2.45) the predicted line width at 77°K is about 0·03 gauss. Since the observed line widths at this temperature are between 2·5 and 3·5 gauss, some other line broadening process is dominant at low temperatures, where the phonon-induced relaxation process is ineffective.

If the line width at 77°K is subtracted from the line widths at higher temperatures, then the resultant curves lie fairly close to a $T^{5/2}$ temperature-dependence.

A complicating factor in this temperature range is that

inter-valley scattering, via Umklapp processes,* to the opposite valley may be an effective relaxation mechanism.[27,28] As the conduction-band minima lie 15 per cent in from the zone boundary in the (100) directions, the wave vector of the longitudinal phonons involved must lie near $q = 0.30\ q_{max}$ (i.e. $q = 0.35 \times 10^8\ cm^{-1}$). Thus this interaction would become effective for $T > 160°K$, since the velocity of sound in the [100] direction is $5.9 \times 10^3\ msec^{-1}$.

The source of the observed line width at temperatures below 77°K is not yet clearly understood. The line broadening mechanism may be some form of impurity scattering process[24] or may be incompletely averaged-out hyperfine structure. Kodera[29,30] has investigated the effect of donor-impurity concentration on the conduction electron resonance in phosphorus-doped silicon and has concluded that the width is related to impurity band conduction.

§2.5

RELAXATION TIMES OF BOUND ELECTRONS IN
PHOSPHOROUS-DOPED SILICON

The spin-lattice relaxation times, at low temperatures, of the donor electrons, are unusually long for electronic relaxation times and have rapidly attracted considerable attention. Relaxation times of the order of 1000 sec have been observed in phosphorus-doped silicon.

In the field of E.S.R. as a whole, the agreement between the theory of relaxation processes and the observed relaxation times is not as good as might be desired. There are usually several competing relaxation processes in any given situation and considerable experimental ingenuity is required to study one process alone. Even then, the effect of defects of various types in the crystal lattices, and of non-stochiometry, make difficult the close comparison of theory and experiment.

---

* *Umklapp processes.* Electron-phonon scattering processes for which

$$k' = k \pm q + 2\pi b$$

are called Umklapp processes, where k, k' are the intitial and final electron wave vectors respectively, q is the wave vector of the emitted or absorbed phonon and b is a reciprocal lattice vector. In cubic crystals $2\pi b = 2\pi/a \cdot n$, where n is a vector with integral components.

So for inter-valley scattering $|q| = 2\pi/a - 2k_0$, where k_0 is the electron wave vector at the conduction-band minimum.

Now in silicon $k_0 = 0.85(\pi/a)$ and so $|q| = 0.30\ (\pi/a)$.

Phosphorus-doped silicon has been the subject of intensive theoretical and experimental investigations since the host crystal can be produced in the form of good, very pure, single crystals. Also the energy-level system of the phosphorus centre is comparatively simple (see Fig. 6.2). As $I = \frac{1}{2}$ for P^{31}, there are no complications from quadrupole effects. Even so, residual impurities and local strains are thought to be responsible for discrepancies in the results obtained by different workers.

It is useful to write down the thermal equilibrium populations of the four-level system of phosphorus-doped silicon. We have, for a given m_I

$$n(+\tfrac{1}{2}) = n(-\tfrac{1}{2}) \exp(-2\Delta) \tag{2.46}$$

where $n(+\frac{1}{2})$ refers to the condition where $m_s = +\frac{1}{2}$ and $2\Delta = g_B H/kT$, and it is assumed that $g_N \beta_N \ll g\beta$, and $a \ll g\beta H$.

Whence, if N is the concentration of phosphorus atoms

$$n(+\tfrac{1}{2}) = \frac{N}{4}(1 - \Delta)$$

$$n(-\tfrac{1}{2}) = \frac{N}{4}(1 + \Delta) \tag{2.47}$$

In Fig. 6.2 are shown the populations of the levels and three relaxation processes, the latter being characterized by the selection rules

$$T_s: \quad \Delta m_s = \pm 1 \qquad \Delta m_I = 0$$

$$T_N: \quad \Delta m_s = 0 \qquad \Delta m_I = \pm 1 \tag{2.48}$$

$$T_x: \quad \Delta m_s = \pm 1 \qquad \Delta m_I = \pm 1$$

Despite the simplicity of the energy-level system the problem of elucidating the various relaxation processes is very complicated. For phosphorus concentrations below 10^{16} cm^{-3} approximately, T_s is independent of the phosphorus concentration and $T_s \propto T^{-1}$ for $T < 2°$K; $-T_s \propto T^{-7}$ for $2°$K $< T < 4.2°$K. T_s is proportional to H^{-4} ($H \geqslant 3000$ gauss) in the temperature range where it is proportional to T^{-1}. Additionally T_s is very dependent on the phosphorus content for concentrations greater than 10^{16} cm^{-3}, falling to 10^{-4} sec at 3×10^{17} phosphorus atoms

per cm^{-3}. In this concentration-dependent region, T_s is sensitive
to the concentration of compensating acceptor centres in the
material.

Also, T_s is reduced in samples exposed to light and in fact care
has to be taken to shield the sample from the background black-
body radiation transmitted along the waveguide from the waveguide components which are at room temperature. The effect of
the light is to excite electrons into the conduction band from the
valence band, or from the donor levels, and these conduction
electrons can relax the donor electrons via a spin-exchange
process.

Following the early experimental work, Pines, Bardeen and
Slichter[31] carried out a detailed study of many possible electron-
spin relaxation processes.

Lattice vibrations modulate both the donor-electron spin-
orbit coupling and the hyperfine interaction between the donor
electron and the donor-impurity nucleus. Thus time-dependent
terms are introduced into the Hamiltonian (equation 2.1), and
can cause transitions between the spin-states.

By considering the effect on the g-factor of uniform dilations
only, Pines, Bardeen, and Slichter obtained $T_s \geqslant 4{\cdot}5 \times 10^3$ sec,
although more detailed work by Abrahams[32] gave a value of
$\sim 10^9$ sec. A relaxation time of this magnitude cannot be observed
in practice.

Modulation of the hyperfine coupling between the donor electron
and the donor-impurity nucleus, by lattice vibrations, can cause
mutual spin flips and hence cause a T_x relaxation process (Fig. 6.2).
By considering the effect of a uniform dilation of the lattice upon
the hyperfine coupling, Pines, Bardeen, and Slichter found

$$T_x \propto (\nu_0 a)^{-2}(IT)^{-1} \qquad (2.49)$$

where a is the hyperfine coupling constant, I is the nuclear spin
and ν_0 is the microwave frequency at resonance. At $\nu_0 = 9$ Gc/s
and $T = 1{\cdot}2°$K, the calculated magnitude of T_x is 9 hours approximately. The modulation of the hyperfine coupling between the
donor electron and the Si^{29} nuclei by lattice vibrations was also
considered, but the calculated values for T_s were greater than 1000
hours and hence this process could not compete with those
considered above.

Concentration-independent region

Feher and Gere[33] have carried out a beautiful series of experiments on phosphorus-doped silicon in both the concentration-independent and concentration-dependent regions. The experiments were designed to study separately the various competing relaxation processes in the light of the available theories.

The T_s process, which is faster than T_x, can be studied by inverting the populations of the levels by 'adiabatic fast passage' through the resonance magnetic field. By monitoring the E.S.R. signal, as the spin system relaxes to the thermal equilibrium distribution, the relaxation time can be calculated from

$$(N_+ - N_-) = (N_+ - N_-)_0 \left[1 - \exp(-t/T_s) \right] \qquad (2.50)$$

where $(N_+ - N_-)_0$ is the difference of populations of the levels at thermal equilibrium.

Honig and Stupp[34] and Feher and Gere[33] found $T_s \propto T^{-1}$ for temperatures between $1\cdot25°$K and $2°$K and $T_s \propto T^{-7}$ between $3°$K and $4°$K. In addition, Honig and Stupp[35] observed $T_s \propto H^4$ for H above 8000 gauss, but a weaker dependence at lower fields was attributed to the contribution of a field independent relaxation process.

The T_s relaxation process in the concentration-independent region is of basic interest. Roth[7] and Hasegawa[8] have calculated T_s for a one-phonon process due to modulation of the electron spin-orbit coupling by lattice vibrations.

Since the g-value of the donor electron is anisotropic, it is expected that there will be an interaction between the electron spin and shear waves, and this will cause relaxation of the spin system.

Two effects of an applied stress, namely the valley-repopulation and one-valley effects, which gave rise to g-shifts were described on pp. 26 to 30. Hence we expect there to be a relaxation process associated with each of these effects.

According to Roth[7] and Hasegawa[8] the spin-lattice relaxation time for the valley-repopulation effect for a one-phonon process is given by

$$\frac{1}{T_s} = \frac{1}{90\pi} \left(\frac{g_\parallel - g_\perp}{g_0} \right)^2 \left(\frac{D_u}{E_{12}} \right)^2 \left(\frac{1}{\rho \bar{V}_2^5} + \frac{2}{3\rho \bar{V}_1^5} \right) \left(\frac{g_0 \beta H}{\hbar} \right)^4$$
$$\times (kT) \sin^2\theta (1 + 3 \cos^2\theta) \qquad (2.51)$$

where ρ is the density of silicon, $\bar{V}_2$ is the velocity of the transverse mode $(5 \cdot 42 \times 10^5$ cm sec$^{-1})$, $\bar{V}_1$ is the velocity of the longitudinal mode $(9 \cdot 33 \times 10^5$ cm sec$^{-1})$ and θ is the angle between the magnetic field and the [100] direction.

For the one-valley effect, the predicted relaxation time for a one-phonon process is given by

$$\frac{1}{T_s} = \frac{1}{20\pi}\left(\frac{A}{g_0}\right)^2\left(\frac{1}{\rho\bar{V}_2{}^5} + \frac{2}{3\rho\bar{V}_1{}^5}\right)\left(\frac{g_0\beta H}{\hbar}\right)^4$$
$$\times (kT)x(\cos^4\theta + \tfrac{1}{2}\sin^4\theta) \qquad (2.52)$$

where $A = 0 \cdot 44$ [see §2.3(b)]. x is defined in §2.3(a).

The valley-repopulation and one-valley effects cannot be separated experimentally. Wilson and Feher[10] fitted the sum of two curves with the angular dependences of equations (2.51) and (2.52) to their experimental results for the angular variation of the one-phonon relaxation time. From the required normalization the calculated relaxation rates for H in the [111] direction were

Valley-repopulation

$$\frac{1}{T_s} = 1 \cdot 1 \times 10^{-3} \text{ sec}^{-1} \qquad (2.53)$$

One-valley

$$\frac{1}{T_s} = 0 \cdot 3 \times 10^{-3} \text{ sec}^{-1} \qquad (2.54)$$

The values for T_s predicted by equations (2.51) and (2.52) are about twice as long as the observed values.

For the Raman (two-phonon) process Roth[7] obtained $(T_s)^{-1} \propto H^2T^7$, but the predicted magnitude of T_s at $4 \cdot 2°$K was 60 sec, compared with the experimentally observed value of 25 sec.[33]

The quartic magnetic field dependence predicted for the one-phonon process by equation (2.51) has been observed experimentally for $H > 8000$ gauss.[35] The quadratic magnetic field dependence predicted for the Raman process has not been observed experimentally.

A good example of the type of experimental technique used to study a particular relaxation process in the presence of others is afforded by the measurement of T_x. Since $T_x \gg T_s$, the short-circuiting effect of the T_s process has to be eliminated. The

4

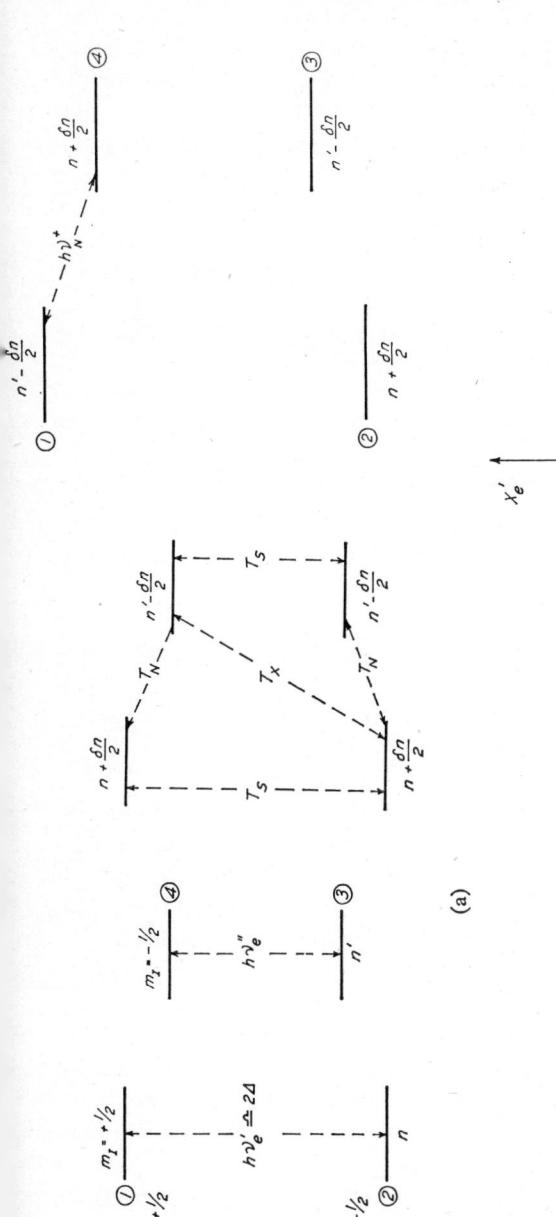

(a)

(b)

Fig. 2.5. Measurement of T_z in phosphorus-doped silicon. (a) The 1–2 and 3–4 microwave transitions are maintained in the saturated condition long enough for the T_z relaxation process to establish a significant population difference between levels 2 and 4. (b) The saturating microwave field is turned off and the population of levels 1 and 4 are inverted by adiabatic fast passage through the radio frequency transition $h\nu_{N+}$. The E.S.R. spectrum now shows one emission and one absorption line, whose amplitudes are a function of the time the T_z relaxation process is allowed to proceed.

experimental procedure is as follows (see Fig. 2.5). The populations of levels 1 and 2, 3 and 4 are equalized by saturating the two
hyperfine lines, the saturating microwave power being switched
off as the magnetic field is swept through the value corresponding
to the 2–4 transition. The 1–2 and 3–4 transitions are maintained
in the saturated state long enough for the T_x process to establish a significant population difference between 2 and 4 (since
$T_s \sim 1000$ sec, the 1–2 and 3–4 transitions do not 'desaturate'
significantly between successive sweeps of the magnetic field).

In the saturated condition, and before the T_x process has
significantly altered the relative populations, we have, referring to
Fig. 2.5,

$$2n + 2n' = N \tag{2.55}$$

and, neglecting the nuclear interaction energy, we have

$$\frac{n'}{n} \simeq (1 - 2\Delta) \tag{2.56}$$

Thus

$$n \simeq \frac{N}{4}(1 + \Delta) \tag{2.57}$$

and

$$n' \simeq \frac{N}{4}(1 - \Delta) \tag{2.58}$$

After the T_x process has significantly altered these populations,
we have the situation shown in Fig. 2.5(*b*). Now the populations
of 1 and 4 are inverted by an adiabatic fast passage through the
nuclear transition $h\nu_N{}^+$, with the saturating microwave power
switched off. If the E.S.R. is now monitored, one emission and
one absorption line are obtained as shown in Fig. 2.5(*b*). Thus, by
measuring the amplitudes as a function of the time for which the
T_x process is allowed to proceed, and knowing the amplitude
of the lines corresponding to the thermal equilibrium situation,
T_x can be calculated. Feher and Gere[33] found $T_x \simeq 30$ hours for
$H = 3200$ gauss and $T_x \simeq 5$ hours for $H \simeq 8000$ gauss, both
results being obtained at $1 \cdot 25°$K.

The magnetic field dependence of the relaxation processes can be
measured by allowing the 'disturbed' populations to relax at the
desired magnetic field for a convenient time. Subsequently, the

magnetic field is returned to the appropriate value for the microwave spectrometer employed and the E.S.R. signal monitored in
the usual way.

Since the relaxation times encountered are so long, no significant
errors are introduced during the time which must necessarily
elapse while the magnetic field is being changed.

The lower limit for T_N has been found to be 10 hours.[33]

Concentration-dependent region

For a phosphorus concentration $> 10^{16}$ cm^{-3}, T_s was concentration dependent and was also observed to be independent of the
magnetic field ($T = 1\cdot25°$K; 3000 gauss $< H < 8000$ gauss).
Thus a simple one-phonon process seems to be ruled out. The
relaxation time T_s is also dependent on the degree of compensation
of the sample, i.e. on the concentration of acceptor impurities.
Feher and Gere[33] observed that the relaxation rate $1/T_s$ was greatest
for the most highly compensated sample ($1\cdot25°$K $< T < 4\cdot2°$K),
and that it was not a simple function of temperature.[33] The
acceptor states are 'filled' by electrons from the donor states and
hence there is a concentration of 'empty' donors equal to the concentration of acceptor impurities. The remaining donor electrons
may 'hop' to an empty donor centre (this is the basis of one kind of
impurity conduction process[18,19]) and this may affect the relaxation time. No theory has as yet been put forward to describe this
effect successfully.

It has been suggested that, in this concentration-dependent
region, spin diffusion to close pairs of donor impurities, which
themselves are fast relaxing centres, is the dominant T_s process.[32]

The spin-lattice relaxation time is very much reduced in samples
exposed to light (this is true of the concentration-independent
region as well). It is thought that some form of exchange process,
in which the optically produced conduction electrons and the
bound donor electrons exchange places, is responsible for the
reduction in T_s. The conduction electrons are then assumed to
relax via some spin-lattice interaction. However, as there will
typically be only $\sim 10^6$ conduction electrons available to relax
$\sim 10^{16}$ donor electrons, there will be a 'bottleneck' in the relaxation
process unless the spin-lattice relaxation time of the conduction

electrons $\lesssim 10^{-9}$ sec, which is much shorter than the observed times.

However, it was pointed out[33] that a double spin exchange mechanism which results in a donor electron moving to another donor with a different nuclear spin orientation, and flipping its own spin in the process, can remove the bottleneck. This is called a T_{ss} process and T_{ss} was found to be 1 sec in a sample having $N_d \simeq 4 \times 10^{16}$ cm^{-3} (number of conduction electrons $\simeq 4 \times 10^6$ cm^{-3}), as compared with $T_s = 25$ sec.

It can be seen that extreme care has to be taken to exclude light and room-temperature radiation from the sample when investigating the long relaxation times in the concentration-independent region. Room-temperature radiation from the waveguide components can be excluded by inserting a glass window in the waveguide and the cavity can be wrapped in a suitable shroud to exclude light.

§2.6

RELAXATION PROCESSES IN ANTIMONY-, ARSENIC- AND
BISMUTH-DOPED SILICON

Arsenic-doped silicon

Measurements of the relaxation times T_s and T_x have been made in arsenic-doped silicon by Culvahouse and Pipkin.[36]

For stable As^{75} ($2 \cdot 8 \times 10^{16}$ atoms cm^{-3}), the measured value of T_s was 390 ± 60 sec and of T_x was 282 ± 60 sec. An irradiated specimen containing 3×10^{10} atoms cm^{-3} of the unstable, 27-hour, As^{76} ($I = 1$) nuclei was also investigated. Polarization of the As^{76} nuclei was produced by saturating a so-called forbidden transition $[\Delta(m_s + m_I) = 0]$ and detected by observing the anisotropy of the emitted γ-rays.[36,37] For As^{76} it was found that $T_s = 240 \pm 120$ sec and $T_x \geqslant 4 \cdot 5 \times 10^3$ sec. From their results Culvahouse and Pipkin found $a_{75} = 197 \cdot 6 \pm 0 \cdot 5$ Mc/s and $a_{76} = -93 \cdot 6 \pm 0 \cdot 5$ Mc/s, and hence $g_{76} = -0 \cdot 453 \pm 0 \cdot 002$, i.e. the nuclear magnetic moment of As^{76} is negative. Equation (2.49) predicts

$$\frac{T_x^{76}}{T_x^{75}} = \frac{I_{75}}{I_{76}} \left(\frac{a_{75}}{a_{76}}\right)^2 \simeq 3 \qquad (2.59)$$

whereas the experiments yielded for this ratio a value of approximately 16.

The temperature dependence of T_s and valley-orbit splittings

In certain situations the maximum phonon energy is greater than the splitting of the low-lying excited states above the ground state. Orbach[38] has considered this kind of situation, with particular reference to the rare earth ions in crystals, and found that relaxation could take place via resonant absorption and emission of phonons between the ground state and low-lying excited states. This kind of situation also exists in silicon containing shallow donor impurities, where the splitting of the doublet/triplet state from the singlet ground state is $\sim 10^{-2}$ eV. The expression obtained by Orbach for the spin-lattice relaxation time is of the form

$$T_s^{-1} = R \exp(-\Delta E/kT) \qquad (2.60)$$

where R is the rate constant for the process and ΔE is the energy splitting to the first excited state ($\Delta E = E_{12}$ in silicon). A phonon with $\hbar w_q \simeq E_{12}$ is absorbed by the donor impurity, exciting the donor electron into the doublet/triplet level, where there is a small, but finite, probability of a spin-flip occurring before the electron returns to the ground state.

Castner[27,28] has measured T_s in antimony-, phosphorus-, arsenic-, and bismuth-doped silicon over the range of temperature 2·5°K to 33°K, and compared his results with the empirical expression

$$T_s^{-1} = AH^4T + BH^2T^7 + CT^9 + DT^{13} + R \cdot \exp-\left(\frac{E_{12}}{kT}\right) \quad (2.61)$$

Here the various terms relate to different postulated relaxation processes. At low temperatures the linear dependence of T_s^{-1} on temperature was observed ('direct' process), at intermediate temperatures a magnetic field independent T^n dependence (with n nearer to 9 than to 7), and at high temperatures an exponential temperature dependence (see Fig. 2.6). The transitions between the various regimes occur at different temperatures for the different donor impurities. For phosphorus, antimony, arsenic and bismuth the transition to the exponential regime was observed by Castner to be at 6°K, approximately 4°K, 11°K and 26°K, respectively.

From the slopes of the graphs of $\log T_s$ versus T^{-1}, in the

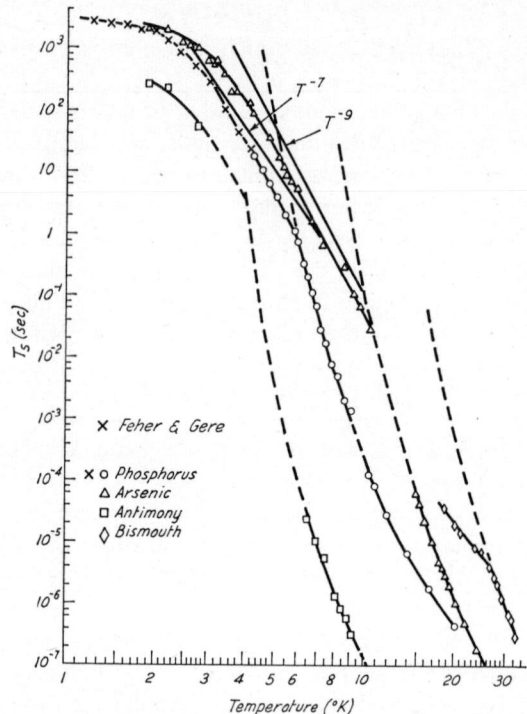

FIG. 2.6. Spin-lattice relaxation time T_s versus temperature for donor-impurity atoms in silicon showing the different temperature dependences. (After Castner.[27])

'exponential' region, Castner was able to measure E_{12} directly for the various donor impurities. By using the observed values of the optical ionization energies, the energy of the first excited level (the doublet/triplet) can be calculated, the results being shown in Table 2.3. The energy of the doublet/triplet level is essentially the same for all the donor-impurity centres and is in good agreement with the value predicted by the effective mass theory. In fact the experimental value for the energy lies slightly below that given by the effective mass theory and this discrepancy is ascribed to the breakdown of the concept of a dielectric constant at small distances from the donor nucleus: the greater the dielectric constant the 'shallower' the donor levels.

TABLE 2.3 Valley-orbit splittings and deformation potentials in silicon

Donor impurity	E_{12}/D_u (×10³)	$E_{12}^{(a)}$ (×10³ eV)	$E_{12}^{(b)}$ (×10³ eV)	Double/Triplet energy,(b) E' (×10³ eV)	Rate constant,(b) R (×10⁻¹⁰ sec⁻¹)	Deformation potential,(c) D_u (eV)
Sb	1·10±0·07	12	9·1±0·3	−33·5	26	8·3
P	1·32±0·08	15	10·6±0·2	−34	{0·091, 0·020}	8·0
As	1·98±0·12	22	19·8±0·4	−33·6	{6·4, 1·5}	10·0
Bi			34±2	−36·0	52	

(a) Taken from Wilson and Feher.[10]   (b) Taken from Castner.[28]   (c) Taken from Castner.[27]

By making use of the values for D_u/E_{12} measured by Wilson and Feher,[10] Castner calculated values for D_u (see Table 2.3). The rate constant, R, for the Orbach process seems to be strongly dependent on the atomic number of the donor impurity and Castner[28] suggests that the spin-flip mechanism may be related to the spin-orbit coupling of the impurity.

§2.7

LITHIUM-DOPED SILICON

Lithium forms a shallow donor centre with an ionization energy of 0·033 eV when diffused into silicon. The experimental evidence suggests that the lithium atoms enter the silicon lattice in interstitial positions and that the donor centre is in fact a lithium-oxygen pair. Oxygen is incorporated into the silicon during the crystal-growing process and its concentration may be $\sim 10^{18}$ atoms cm^{-3}.

Honig and Kip[39] observed a single E.S.R. line ($g = 1 \cdot 999$) in a lithium-doped silicon sample with $N_d = 7 \times 10^{16}$ cm^{-3}. The experiments were carried out at 8800 Mc/s and 300 Mc/s. The line was inhomogeneously broadened, i.e. there was unresolved hyperfine structure.

A small asymmetry of the resonance line prompted further experiments at higher frequencies (K band), which revealed a pair of lines whose relative position and intensity varied with the orientation of the sample with respect to the applied magnetic field.[5] These results can be described by an axially symmetric **g**-tensor, the symmetry axis being in the [111] crystal direction. This model predicts that, for H in the [100] direction, all four [111] directions are equivalent and a single resonance line should be observed. For H applied in the [111] direction, two lines, with an intensity ratio of 3 : 1, and having g-values of $g_\perp$ and $g_\parallel$ respectively, are expected. For H in the [110] direction, two lines of equal amplitude are predicted (see Fig. 2.7). The measured g-values are $g_\parallel = 1 \cdot 9978 \pm 0 \cdot 0001$ and $g_\perp = 1 \cdot 9992 \pm 0 \cdot 0001$.

The hyperfine interaction with the lithium nucleus can be resolved by using the E.N.D.O.R. technique. Feher found $a(Li^7) = 0 \cdot 845 \pm 0 \cdot 003$ Mc/s, which gives

$$|\Psi(0)|^2 = 0 \cdot 33 \times 10^{22} \, cm^{-3}$$

compared with a theoretical value of 0.2×10^{22} cm^{-3}. He also investigated a sample enriched with Li^6 and found

$$a(\text{Li}^6) = 0.316 \pm 0.001 \text{ Mc/s}.$$

§2.8

SHALLOW ACCEPTOR IMPURITIES

The acceptor wave functions are built up from Bloch functions chosen from near the valence-band maximum but, since the valence band is six-fold degenerate (including spin) near $k = 0$, the situation is more complicated than for donor impurities

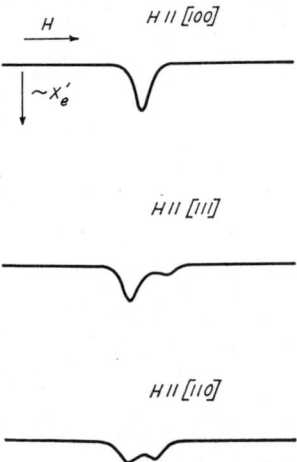

FIG. 2.7. E.S.R. spectrum of lithium-doped silicon ($\sim 3 \times 10^{16}$ Li atoms cm^{-3}) at $1.25°$K, using a microwave frequency in the region of 22 700 Mc/s. The splitting is due to an anisotropic g-value and this indicates that the donor-electron wave function does not have tetrahedral symmetry. (After Feher.[5])

(see §1.4). Local strains (due to dislocations and impurities for instance) cause a splitting of the $j = \frac{3}{2}$ band by random amounts $\delta E = D_v S_i$, where D_v is the deformation potential for the valence band and S_i the local strain.[3,40]

Feher *et al.*[41] found that spin resonance of holes bound to acceptor impurities could only be observed if the silicon sample was subjected to a uniaxial stress in the region of 900 kg cm^{-2}. This observation was interpreted as follows. For zero externally applied stress, $D_v S_i \gtrsim g_A \beta H$ and hence m_J is not a good quantum number, i.e. the wave functions for the four states into which the $J = \frac{3}{2}$ band splits, because of the effect of local strains and an applied magnetic field, are mixtures of 'pure' m_J functions. In this situation

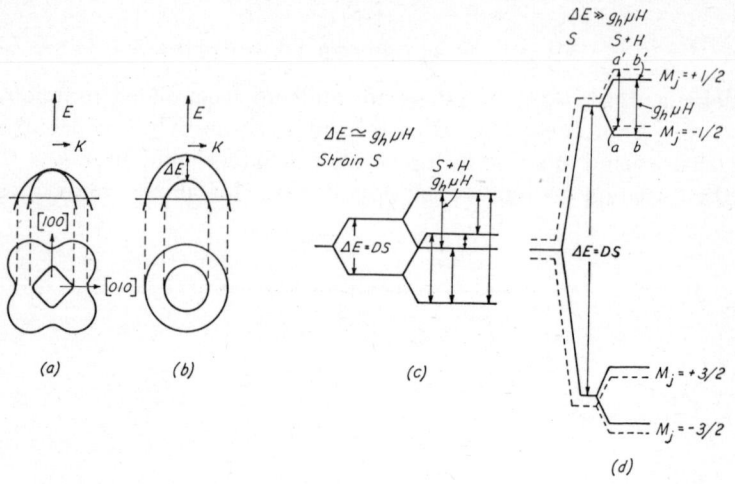

Fig. 2.8. Valence band in silicon.
(*a*) In the absence of stress.   (*b*) With applied uniaxial stress.
(*c*) Energy levels with $\Delta E \simeq g_h \mu H$. All six transitions indicated are allowed. The resonance line will be broadened and difficult to observe.
(*d*) Energy levels with $\Delta E \gg g_h \mu H$. The transition frequencies are $aa' = bb'$. Lines will not be broadened by random internal strains and paramagnetic resonance is observable.
(By courtesy of G. Feher *et al.*[41])

all six spin transitions are allowed (see Fig. 2.8) and this fact, combined with the randomness of the local strains, produces line broadening such that resonance cannot be observed. If, however, a large strain S_{ext} is produced by an externally applied stress, such that $D_v S_{ext} \gg D_v S_i$ and $g_A \beta H$, then m_J becomes a good quantum number and local strains do not broaden the resonance. From measurements of the anisotropy of the transition probability Feher *et al.* deduced that, even under the large stresses applied, the states were not pure m_J states.

Spin resonance has been observed for the shallow acceptor impurities B, Al, Ga and In and for the deep-lying impurity

Zn^-.[42,43] Feher *et al.*[41] found that for boron, which has the smallest binding energy of the shallow acceptor impurities, $g_\parallel = 1.21 \pm 0.01$ and $g_\perp = 2.43 \pm 0.01$; this is in excellent agreement with the prediction of Luttinger[44] that $g_\perp/g_\parallel = 2$ for free holes in the valence band.

It is possible for two species of spins having different g-values to interact at a value of the magnetic field so that the resonance lines overlap. For instance, in silicon containing phosphorus and iron, such a resonant spin-spin interaction occurs for the $m_I = +\frac{1}{2}$ line when the following condition is satisfied:[33]

$$g_P \beta H_M + \frac{a}{2} = g_{Fe} \beta H_M \qquad (2.62)$$

The 'mixing' field H_M has a value of about 600 gauss. Since the spin-lattice relaxation time for the iron is much shorter than that of the phosphorus centres, it is possible to observe the resonant spin-spin interaction in the following way. Both spin systems are allowed to come to thermal equilibrium with the lattice at $1.25°K$ in a field ~ 3000 gauss. The spin systems are now allowed to mix at $H \simeq 600$ gauss for a time much greater than $T_s(Fe)$ but much less than $T_s(P)$. Hence, on monitoring the phosphorus spin resonance spectrum at 9 KMc/s, the $m_I = +\frac{1}{2}$ line is much less intense than the $m_I = -\frac{1}{2}$ line, since the intensity of the latter corresponds to a Boltzmann factor for $H \sim 3000$ gauss, whereas the former corresponds to a Boltzmann factor for $H \simeq 600$ gauss.

Levy[45] was able to measure the g-value for acceptors in a compensated *n*-type sample of silicon (5×10^{15} phosphorus atoms cm^{-3} and 3×10^{15} boron atoms cm^{-3}) by observing the reduction of the relaxation time of the donor electrons on the phosphorus atoms. The relaxation time was due to resonant spin-spin interaction with the broad acceptor resonance. Under conditions of zero externally applied stress, the $m_I = -\frac{1}{2}$ line relaxed fastest. H_M can be determined by noting the value of mixing field which gives the maximum difference in amplitude for the two phosphorus hyperfine lines. The energy difference for the $m_I = -\frac{1}{2}$ donor-electron transition is given by the Breit-Rabi formula[46] (see §6.5) and is

$$\Delta E_D = -\frac{a}{2}[-1 + x + (1 + x^2)^{1/2}] \qquad (2.63)$$

where $x \equiv 2\beta H/a$. The nuclear Zeeman interaction has been neglected and the g-value of the donor resonance has been assumed to be 2.

For the acceptor resonance, the energy difference may be written as

$$\Delta E_A = g_A a x/2 \qquad (2.64)$$

Equating (2.63) and (2.64) we have

$$g_A = [-1 + x + (1 + x^2)^{1/2}]/x \qquad (2.65)$$

Levy obtained $g_A \simeq 1\cdot 6$ in an unstrained crystal where, of course, it is difficult to find H_M precisely. In a uniaxially strained crystal ($250\ \mathrm{kgm/cm^2}$), the $m_I = +\frac{1}{2}$ line was observed to have the shorter relaxation time and the value of g_A was $2\cdot 43 \pm 0\cdot 6$, which compares well with an extrapolated value of $2\cdot 39$ obtained from Feher's measurements.

The spin-lattice relaxation rate of boron has been measured by Ludwig and Woodbury,[42] and Shimizu and Nakayama.[47] It was found to be extremely stress-dependent, becoming very large for small strains.

References

1. Portis, A. M., Kip, A. F., Kittel, C., and Brattain, W. H., *Phys. Rev.*, 1953, **90**, 488.
2. Fletcher, R. C., Yager, W. A., Pearson, G. L., Holden, A. N., Read, W. T., and Merritt, F. R., *Phys. Rev.*, 1954, **94**, 1392.
3. Kohn, W., *Solid State Physics*, Vol. 5, p. 258 (Academic Press Inc., 1957).
4. Fletcher, R. C., Yager, W. A., Pearson, G. L., and Merritt, F. R., *Phys. Rev.*, 1954, **95**, 944.
5. Feher, G., *Phys. Rev.*, 1959, **114**, 1219.
6. Feher, G., *Phys. Rev.*, 1958, **109**, 221.
7. Roth, L. M., *Phys. Rev.*, 1960, **118**, 1534.
8. Hasegawa, H., *Phys. Rev.*, 1960, **118**, 1523.
9. Kohn, W., *Solid State Physics*, Vol. 5, p. 257 (Academic Press Inc., 1957).
10. Wilson, D. K., and Feher, G., *Phys. Rev.*, 1961, **124**, 1068.
11. Liu, L., *Phys. Rev.*, 1962, **126**, 1317.
12. Kohn, W., and Luttinger, J. M., *Phys. Rev.*, 1955, **98**, 915.
13. Kittel, C., *Introduction to Solid State Physics*, 2nd ed., Chapter 4 (John Wiley & Sons Inc., 1960).
14. Yafet, Y., *Solid State Physics*, Vol. 14, p. 90 (Academic Press Inc., 1963).
15. Lancaster, G., and Schneider, E. E., *Proceedings of the International Conference on Semiconductor Physics*, p. 589 (Czech. Acad. of Sci., 1961).
16. Walters, G. K., *J. Phys. Chem. Solids (GB)*, 1960, **14**, 43.
17. Dyson, F. J., *Phys. Rev.*, 1955, **98**, 349.

18. Mott, N. F., and Twose, W. D., *Adv. in Physics*, 10, No. 38, p. 107 (1961).
19. Miller, A., and Abrahams, E., *Phys. Rev.*, 1960, **120**, 745.
20. Slichter, C. P., *Phys. Rev.*, 1955, **99**, 479.
21. See for instance: Schiff, L. I., *Quantum Mechanics* (McGraw-Hill, 1955).
22. Lancaster, G., van Wyk, J. A., Schneider, E. E., *Proc. Phys. Soc.*, 1964, **84**, 19.
23. Gere, E. A., Bell Telephone Laboratories Internal Report.
24. Pines, D., and Slichter, C. P., *Phys. Rev.*, 1955, **100**, 1014.
25. Wangsness, R. K., and Bloch, F., *Phys. Rev.*, 1953, **89**, 728.
26. Elliott, R. J., *Phys. Rev.*, 1954, **96**, 266.
27. Castner, T. G., *Phys. Rev. Letters*, 1962, **8**, 13.
28. Castner, T. G., *Phys. Rev.*, 1963, **130**, 58.
29. Kodera, H., *J. Phys. Soc. Japan*, 1964, **19**, 915.
30. Kodera, H., *J. Phys. Soc. Japan*, 1964, **19**, 1751.
31. Pines, D., Bardeen, J., and Slichter, C. P., *Phys. Rev.*, 1957, **106**, 489.
32. Abrahams, E., *Phys. Rev.*, 1957, **107**, 491.
33. Feher, G., and Gere, E. A., *Phys. Rev.*, 1959, **114**, 1245.
34. Honig, A., and Stupp, E., *Phys. Rev.*, 1960, **117**, 69.
35. Honig, A., and Stupp, E., *Phys. Rev. Letters*, 1958, **1**, 275.
36. Culvahouse, J. W., and Pipkin, F. M., *Phys. Rev.*, 1957, **106**, 1102.
37. Jeffries, C. D., *Phys. Rev.*, 1957, **106**, 164.
38. Orbach, R., *Proc. Phys. Soc.*, 1960, **77**, 821.
39. Honig, A., and Kip, A. F., *Phys. Rev.*, 1954, **95**, 1686.
40. Bir, G. L., Butikov, E. I., Pikus, G. E., *J. Phys. Chem. Solids (GB)*, 1963, **24**, 1467.
41. Feher, G., Hensel, J. C., Gere, E. A., *Phys. Rev. Letters*, 1960, **5**, 309.
42. Ludwig, G. W., Woodbury, H. H., *Bull. Am. Phys. Soc.*, 1961, **6**, 118.
43. Ludwig, G. W., Woodbury, H. H., *Solid State Physics*, Vol. 13, p. 223 (Academic Press Inc., 1962).
44. Luttinger, J. M., *Phys. Rev.*, 1956, **102**, 1030.
45. Levy, R. A., *Phys. Rev. Letters*, 1960, **5**, 425.
46. Breit, G., Rabi, I. I., *Phys. Rev.*, 1940, **38**, 2082.
47. Shimizu, T., Nakayama, M., *J. Phys. Soc. Japan*, 1964, **18**, 1844.

Chapter 3

Deep-Lying States in Silicon

A large number of elements, particularly the transition series ions, give deep levels in the forbidden energy gap when diffused into silicon. Those levels so far observed, and their presumed ionization states, are shown in Fig. 1.4(*a*). Considerable attention has been devoted to the electrical properties of silicon containing these impurity elements,[1] but there is difficulty, in general, in associating observed electrical properties with a specific impurity. There are three principal causes of this difficulty. Firstly, the solubilities of these elements are low (10^{14}–10^{17} atoms cm^{-3}), being of the same order of magnitude as 'accidental' impurities. Secondly, the electrical properties in many cases change with time, presumably owing to precipitation of the impurities. Thirdly, the electrical properties of different impurity elements are similar. The 'diffusion' process is usually carried out at about 1250°C, where the solubilities of the transition metals are at a maximum, and hence, after quenching, the transition metal ion is in a super-saturated solution.

These impurities may exist in different ionization states, and, since these states have relatively high ionization energies, the electrons are localized on the impurity atom and the hydrogen-like effective mass theory cannot be applied. The position in the forbidden energy gap of the Fermi level can be varied by doping with suitable concentrations of shallow donor or acceptor impurities, and various ionization states of the deep-lying levels may be obtained.

It is not possible to determine from electrical measurements what type of site the deep impurities occupy in the crystal or their electronic structures. E.S.R. experiments, carried out notably by G. W. Ludwig, H. H. Woodbury and F. S. Ham, have revealed from the symmetry of the observed spectra, that the transition series ions can occupy substitutional or interstitial sites and may also occur as impurity pairs. Knowledge of these deep-lying impurity centres has been greatly increased by E.S.R. experiments.

§3.1

THE SPIN HAMILTONIAN FOR TRANSITION GROUP IONS IN SILICON

E.S.R. has been observed for several ions of the iron (3d), palladium (4d), and platinum (5d) transition groups of elements (see Table 3.1) and also for impurity pairs, formed generally of a negatively charged substitutional acceptor impurity and a positively charged transition metal ion at a nearest interstitial site.

We have seen in Chapter 2 that for shallow donor impurities the donor electrons are extremely delocalized, and the parameters of the E.S.R. spectrum are determined by the energy-band structure of the host crystal. The resonance properties of the deep-lying impurities have been discussed principally in terms of crystal-field theory, in which the neighbouring ions are treated as point electrical charges, although the effects of covalency have been considered and looked for in E.S.R. spectra. Since the electrons are to a large extent localized on the impurity ion, the total Hamiltonian used is that of the free ion plus terms associated with the effect of the surrounding atoms and ions of the solid. The problem consists of finding the energy levels of the paramagnetic ion in a crystalline field of known symmetry. This approach was developed by Abragam and Pryce[2] and a detailed review has been given by Low.[3] The various orbital levels of the free ion are split by the crystalline electric field, and further splitting may be caused by spin-orbit interaction. Now, in E.S.R. experiments, transitions are observed only between the lowest-lying levels of a paramagnetic ion. The usual approach to interpreting the experimental observations is to treat the levels between which transitions occur as isolated levels and to ignore higher levels. If transitions are observed between $(2J+1)$ levels, then the magnetic behaviour of these low-lying levels is described by means of a spin Hamiltonian,[2,3] which consists of terms containing powers of $\mathbf{H}$, $\mathbf{J}$, and also of $\mathbf{I}$, if the ions of interest have a nuclear magnetic moment. The angular momentum $\mathbf{J}$ has components $\mathbf{S}$ and $\mathbf{L'}$, where $\mathbf{S}$ is the total electron spin of the ion and $\mathbf{L'}$ the effective

TABLE 3.1 Spin resonance results for transition metal ions in silicon[*]

Configuration	Ion	S	J	g	a	Units of 10^{-4} cm^{-1}		
						A	$a_\parallel$	$a_\perp$
Interstitial								
3d^3	$(\text{V}^{51})^{2+}$	3/2	3/2	1·9892		−42·10	2·3	2·3
3d^5	$(\text{Cr}^{53})^{+}$	5/2	5/2	1·9978	+30·16	+10·67	2·2	1·4
	$(\text{Mn}^{55})^{2+}$	5/2	5/2	2·0066	+19·88	−53·47		
3d^6	$(\text{Cr}^{53})^{0}$	2	1	2·97		15·9		
	$(\text{Cr}^{53})^{0}$	2	2	1·72				
3d^7	$(\text{Mn}^{55})^{+}$	2	1	3·01		73·8		
	$(\text{Mn}^{55})^{0}$	3/2	1/2	3·362		92·5		
	$(\text{Mn}^{55})^{0}$	3/2	3/2	1·46				
	$(\text{Fe}^{57})^{+}$	3/2	1/2	3·524		2·99		
3d^8	$(\text{Mn}^{55})^{-}$	1	1	2·0104		−71·28	(∼1)	(∼1)
	$(\text{Fe}^{57})^{0}$	1	1	2·0699		6·98	3	2
3d^9	$(\text{Ni}^{61})^{+}$	1/2	1/2	2·026		3·6	(∼8)	(∼8)
Substitutional								
3d^2	$(\text{Cr}^{53})^{0}$	1	1	1·9962		12·54	17·4	
3d^5	$(\text{Mn}^{55})^{+}$	1	1	2·0259	+26·1	−63·09	9·5	
	$(\text{Mn}^{55})^{2-}$			2·0058		−40·5	4·8	

[*] By courtesy of G. W. Ludwig and H. H. Woodbury,[4] and Academic Press Inc.

orbital angular momentum. Generally, terms containing small powers of $\mathbf{H}$, $\mathbf{J}$, and $\mathbf{I}$ are dominant and for a paramagnetic ion occupying a site having tetrahedral symmetry

$$\mathscr{H} = g\beta \mathbf{J}.\mathbf{H} + \frac{a}{6}(J_x^4 + J_y^4 + J_z^4) + A\mathbf{J}.\mathbf{I} - (g_N + R)\beta_N \mathbf{I}.\mathbf{H} \tag{3.1}$$

Note that, for this site symmetry, g, A, and R are scalar quantities and that the usual zero field splitting term, which has the tensor form $\mathbf{J}.\mathbf{D}.\mathbf{J}$, reduces to a constant, as does the quadruple interaction term $\mathbf{I}.\mathbf{Q}.\mathbf{I}$.[4] In the nuclear Zeeman interaction, R represents an anisotropic term, which, in certain situations, can be as large as the term $g_N\beta_N\mathbf{I}.\mathbf{H}$. From considerations of symmetry, the lowest order term in J (for $J \geqslant 2$) that can give a zero field splitting of the energy levels, is a fourth-order term usually written in the form of the second term of equation (3.1), in which a is the cubic field splitting parameter. Since Si^{29} has a nuclear magnetic moment, the associated hyperfine interaction between the paramagnetic impurity and the 4·7 per cent abundant Si^{29} nucleus has to be included in the spin Hamiltonian, as also has the nuclear Zeeman term. So we must add to equation (3.1) a term of the form

$$\sum_l (\mathbf{J}.\mathscr{A}_l.\mathbf{I}_l - g_l\beta_l\mathbf{I}_l.\mathbf{H}) \tag{3.2}$$

where the sum is over all lattice sites occupied by Si^{29} nuclei. The electron wave function at neighbouring sites does not have tetrahedral symmetry and hence the interaction terms have a tensor form.

In a tetrahedral lattice, the interstitial sites of maximum symmetry lie in $\langle 111 \rangle$ directions from substitutional sites and also have tetrahedral symmetry (see Fig. 3.1). Hence, a spin Hamiltonian of the form (3.1) is applicable to both substitutional and interstitial ions.

The hyperfine interaction depends on the quantity $\langle r^{-3} \rangle$ for the interacting electrons, and if the nuclear magnetic moment is known from other measurements, then $\langle r^{-3} \rangle$ can be measured in the solid. This is of great interest since it yields information on the extent of the electron wave function in the solid and thus gives a measure of covalent bonding.

5

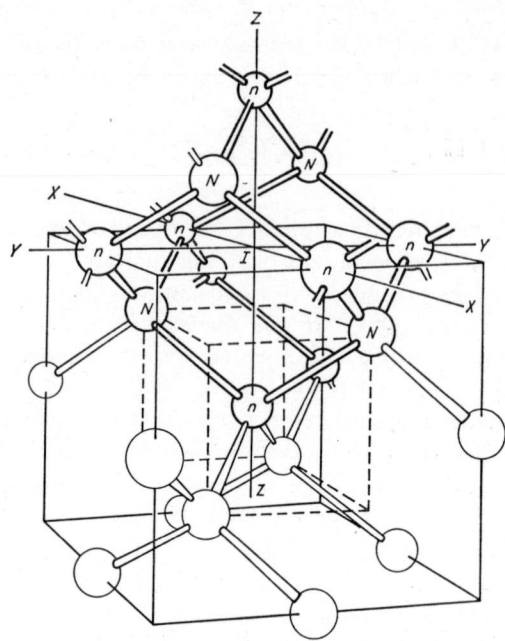

Fɪɢ. 3.1. An interstitial site in the diamond-type lattice, showing the tetrahedrally-arranged nearest neighbours (N) and the octahedrally-arranged nearest neighbours (n).

The E.S.R. spectrum consists of $(2I+1)$ equally spaced hyperfine components, each of which is split into $2J$ fine structure components. Under the usual experimental conditions, the populations of the $(2I+1)$ closely spaced hyperfine levels are very nearly equal, and hence the hyperfine lines are equally intense. This, in principle, enables the hyperfine and fine structure lines to be distinguished apart. However, in practice, line broadening mechanisms may cause either the fine or hyperfine structure to be unresolved.

Several species of impurity pairs have been studied by the E.S.R. and E.N.D.O.R. techniques. Generally, the pairs appear to consist of a negatively charged acceptor ion (of the shallow or deep variety) at a substitutional site, associated with a positively charged transition group ion situated at a nearest interstitial site. A description of the various impurity pairs that have been observed will be given in §3.3. Only the form of the spin Hamiltonian used to describe the spin resonance spectra will be given here.

Ludwig and Woodbury[4] have written the spin Hamiltonian in the form

$$\mathscr{H} = \beta[g_{\parallel}J_zH_z + g_{\perp}(J_xH_x + J_yH_y)] + DJ_z^2$$

$$+ \frac{a}{6}(J_\xi^4 + J_\eta^4 + J_\zeta^4)$$

$$+ \frac{F}{180}[35J_z^4 - 30J(J+1)J_z^2 + 25J_z^2]$$

$$+ \sum_{i=1}^{2}[A_iJ_zI_{i_z} + B_i(J_xI_{i_x} + J_yI_{i_y})]$$

$$+ P_iI_{i_z}^2$$

$$- (\gamma_i + R_{i_{\parallel}})\beta_N I_{i_z}H_z$$

$$- (\gamma_i + R_{i_{\perp}})\beta_N(I_{i_x}H_x + I_{i_y}H_y) \tag{3.3}$$

where the z-axis is taken to be the pair axis. The possibility of hyperfine interactions with both nuclei of the pair is indicated by the sum over subscripts $i = 1, 2$. This spin Hamiltonian reflects the axial symmetry about the pair axis (usually a $\langle 111 \rangle$ direction) and one result is that the g-value is anisotropic (specified by $g_{\parallel}$ and $g_{\perp}$) in contrast with the situation of cubic symmetry where it is isotropic. The main effect of the negatively charged acceptor ion is to introduce non-cubic terms into the crystal potential, which are represented by the terms D, F, and P. Also, the cubic field splitting term is referred to the cubic crystalline axes denoted by ξ, η, ζ.

The observed spectrum in an axially symmetric situation depends on the relative magnitudes of the terms in equation (3.3), particularly the magnitude of the zero field splitting coefficient D with respect to $h\nu$ for the microwave frequency used. If $|2D| \ll h\nu$, $2J$ fine structure lines are observed, each of which is split into hyperfine components, whereas for $|2D| \sim h\nu$ forbidden fine structure transitions ($\Delta m_s = \pm 2$) and forbidden hyperfine transitions ($\Delta m_s = \pm 1$, $\Delta m_I = \pm 1, \pm 2$) may be observed as well.[3,5]

The situation is further complicated for these impurity pairs in that they may be aligned along any of the equivalent $\langle 111 \rangle$ directions (for nearest neighbour pairs). In silicon $|2D| \gtrsim h\nu$ for most of the pairs, although for $(Mn^{55} Pt^{195})$ $|D| > 10 \text{ cm}^{-1}$, i.e. $|2D| \gg h\nu$. Microwave $\Delta m_s = \pm 1$ transitions can only be observed between the $m_s = \pm \frac{1}{2}$ states in this case, owing to the large zero field splitting. Hence, this latter situation has been treated by Ludwig and Woodbury[4] in terms of the following spin Hamiltonian with $J = S' = \frac{1}{2}$:

$$\mathscr{H} = \beta[g_{\shortparallel} S_z' H_z + g_\perp (S_x' H_x + S_y' H_y)]$$
$$+ \sum_{i=1,2} A_i S_z' I_{i_z} + B_i (S_x' I_{i_x} + S_y' I_{i_y}) + P_i I_z^2$$
$$- \beta_N [\gamma_{i_{\shortparallel}} I_{i_z} H_z + \gamma_{i_\perp} (I_{i_x} H_x + I_{i_y} H_y)] \tag{3.4}$$

where

$$\gamma_{i_{\shortparallel}} = \gamma_i + R_{i_{\shortparallel}} \tag{3.5}$$

and

$$\gamma_{i_\perp} = \gamma_i + R_{i_\perp} + g_\perp \left(\frac{B_i}{4D}\right)\left(\frac{\beta}{\beta_N}\right)\left(J - \frac{1}{2}\right)\left(J + \frac{3}{2}\right) \tag{3.6}$$

The method for determining D depends on its magnitude. For $|2D| \ll h\nu$, the value of D can be determined from the fine structure splitting of the ordinary $\Delta m_s = \pm 1$ E.S.R. transitions. For $|2D| \gg h\nu$, we see from equation (3.6) and the spin Hamiltonian (3.4) that D can be determined from E.N.D.O.R. transitions ($\Delta m_s = 0$, $\Delta m_I = \pm 1$). It can also be determined from measurements of the g-value at different microwave frequencies.[5] Another important result of the E.N.D.O.R. experiments is that they have confirmed, from the symmetry of the spectra, that the impurity pairs are aligned in $\langle 111 \rangle$ directions. An exception to this rule appears to be the $(Fe–In)^0$ pair. The symmetry of its E.N.D.O.R. spectrum indicates that it has one impurity atom at a lattice site and the other at a next-nearest interstitial site.

§3.2

EXPERIMENTAL OBSERVATIONS OF TRANSITION GROUP IONS

For ions with $J \leqslant \frac{3}{2}$, the energy levels obtained from equation

(3.1) are

$$W_{m_s, m_I} = g\beta H m_s + A m_s m_I - (g_N + R)\beta_N H m_I$$
$$+ \{m_s[I(I+1) - m_I^2] - m_I[J(J+1) - m_s^2]\} A^2 / 2h\nu$$

(3.7)

If $J \geqslant 2$, the cubic field splitting term must be considered and the fine structure lines are orientation dependent.[3] The situation with $J = \frac{5}{2}$ (Mn^{2+}, Fe^{3+}) is the most important of these cases in silicon.

Vanadium is the least soluble of the iron group ions in silicon (concentration $< 10^{15}$ atoms cm^{-3}). The spectrum shows eight hyperfine components ($I = \frac{7}{2}$ for V^{51}), the $m_I = \pm \frac{7}{2}$ lines of which are split into three fine structure components. Thus it was deduced that $J = \frac{3}{2}$, and this has been confirmed by E.N.D.O.R. experiments.[6] The spectrum has only been observed in low resistivity p-type material. Hence it is thought that two 4s electrons are removed from the free atom electron configuration to fill shallow acceptor states, leaving the impurity ion V^{2+} with the electron configuration 3d^3.

Theory suggests that if chromium is diffused into low resistivity n-type material, it remains electrically neutral (3d^5 4s), while if it is so introduced into p-type silicon, the electron configuration is 3d^5 (Cr^+). Spectra that have been associated with Cr^+ (interstitial) and Cr^0 (both substitutional and interstitial) have been observed. For Cr^+ there are five well-resolved fine structure lines, which have associated with them four weak hyperfine components due to the 9·5 per cent abundant isotope Cr^{53}. For interstitial Cr^0, two fine structure transitions ($\Delta m_s = \pm 1$) are observed, yielding $J = 1$, together with $\Delta m_s = 2$ transitions at half the magnetic field.[4] The spectrum of substitutional Cr^0 is of interest in that the super-hyperfine splitting due to nearest neighbour and next-nearest neighbour Si^{29} (twelve in number for a substitutional site as compared with six for an interstitial site) is resolved. For this substitutional ion, $J = 1$.

E.S.R. spectra have been observed for manganese in four charge states. Isolated impurity atoms are obtained if the silicon sample is rapidly quenched after the diffusion process. Clusters of what are thought to be four manganese ions are formed if the sample is cooled slowly. For isolated interstitial Mn^- ions the fine structure indicates $J = 1$ and this has been confirmed by E.N.D.O.R. experiments. Spin resonance has also been observed for the interstitial manganese ions Mn°, Mn^+, Mn^{2+}. These spectra will be interpreted in terms of the model for the electronic structure of the impurity centres which will be considered in §3.3. Mn^+, which is iso-electronic with Cr^0, can also exist at substitutional sites and its spectrum is similar to that of Cr^0. For the clusters of four manganese ions, twenty-one hyperfine lines corresponding to $\Sigma_{k=1}^{4} m_k$ are observed,[4] and it would seem from the crystal-field splittings of the spectrum that $J = 2$.

Spin resonance from iron has been observed by Feher,[7] and Ludwig and Woodbury.[4,6] The resistivity of n-type material is unchanged when iron is diffused into it and this suggests that, in n-type material, the iron sites are neutral. The absence of a cubic crystal-field splitting implies that $J \leqslant \frac{3}{2}$ and the suggested charge state, having an even number of unpaired electrons, would require J to be integral. If the tetrahedral symmetry is destroyed by applying a uniaxial stress, then two well-resolved fine structure lines are observed,[6] indicating that $J = 1$. This has been confirmed by E.N.D.O.R. experiments. Spin resonance has also been observed for Fe^+.

The only isolated ions of the 4d and 5d transition groups for which E.S.R. has been observed[8] are Pd^- and Pt^-, each of which has a solubility of about 10^{16} atoms cm^{-3}. For both of these ions the impurity site is believed to be distorted in one of the cubic directions. A shift of the axis of symmetry of the Si^{29} hyperfine interaction of about $5°$ away from the $\langle 111 \rangle$ directions is consistent with such a departure from tetrahedral symmetry. For Pt^- an additional spin resonance spectrum has been observed, which may be due to a pair of impurities.

Impurity-pair formation is favoured in samples which are slowly quenched from the diffusion temperature. The principal reasons for this are the fact that interstitial transition group ions are mobile even at $300°K$, and that the interaction energy of such impurities with acceptor impurities is relatively large. Thus, in compensated samples, under equilibrium conditions, there are few isolated impurity ions. Impurity pairs involving chromium, manganese, and iron in association with boron, aluminium, gallium, zinc, indium, gold and platinum have been studied.[4]

By introducing vacancies into silicon containing transition metal ions, it has been possible to determine, with a good degree of certainty, whether ions in various charge states are interstitial or substitutional impurities. The E.S.R. technique has been of particular service in unravelling this problem because of its sensitivity to only those electrically active impurities that are paramagnetic, because of the correlation between the symmetry of the observed spectrum and that of the site of the impurity, and because the number of unpaired electrons may be determined from the number of fine structure lines in the spectrum.

Electrical measurements have shown that whereas the solubility of copper in silicon at the diffusion temperature is about 10^{18} atom cm^{-3}, the concentration of electrically active copper[9] is only about 5×10^{14} atoms cm^{-3}, the difference being accounted for by precipitation. It has been proposed that vacancies generated by the strains set up around precipitates can be produced during the migration of dislocation loops.[10] Alternatively, a reaction of the following type has been proposed:[11]

(substitutional impurity) $\rightarrow$ (interstitial impurity + vacancy)
$\rightarrow$ (precipitate + vacancy)

In rapidly quenched manganese-doped silicon, spin resonance spectra attributed to Mn^- and Mn^{2+} have been observed (see p. 56). If copper and manganese are simultaneously diffused into silicon and the sample is cooled slowly, then for both negative ions in n-type material (excess of phosphorus over compensating impurities) and for positive ions in p-type material (excess of boron over compensating impurities) a new spin resonance spectrum is seen. As both negative ion spectra are seen in silicon containing uncompensated phosphorus, the two species of manganese must be at different sites and cannot be different charge states of one impurity. If manganese alone is diffused into high purity silicon, neither spectrum is seen, and on this basis it is concluded that the difference of the charge states of manganese in the phosphorus- and boron-doped material must be at least two. Further, since there is an even number of unpaired electrons associated with one charge state and an odd number with the other, the difference in charge states must be odd. Hence, Ludwig and Woodbury[11] concluded that the charge states must differ by at least three electrons and postulated Mn^+ and Mn^{2-}, which are the lowest charge states consistent with these conditions. One of these impurity species must be substitutional and the other interstitial since the spin resonance spectra of both exhibit tetrahedral symmetry.

The Mn^+ spectrum in copper-doped samples is much more stable in intensity than that due to Mn^{2+}. Hence it was concluded that Mn^+ is the substitutional species. Similarly, Mn^{2-} is more stable than Mn^-. The ability of manganese in copper-free samples to diffuse and form impurity pairs and clusters of four impurity atoms is additional evidence of manganese being an interstitial impurity.

For the orbitally degenerate ions, the spin-lattice relaxation times are very short and spin resonance cannot be observed above $10°K$. For those ions with an orbital singlet as the ground state, the spin-lattice relaxation time is much longer and spin resonance may be observed up to $78°K$ (for Fe^0).

§3.3

THE ELECTRONIC STRUCTURE OF SUBSTITUTIONAL AND INTERSTITIAL IRON GROUP IONS

In a free atom or ion all five d-orbitals have the same energy, but for an ion in a crystalline electric field this is not so. Group theory is used to solve the problem of determining how this fivefold degeneracy is lifted by the crystalline field. In fact, the most convenient set of linearly-independent, orthogonal, free ion d-functions to use as basis functions have the following spatial dependencies (see Fig. 3.2):

$$xy, yz, zx, x^2 - y^2, 3z^2 - r^2$$

(a common radial factor has been omitted). This set of functions carries a five-dimensional representation of the full rotation group. For an ion in a crystalline electric field having cubic symmetry, these functions split into a group of three and a group of two, carrying the three- and two-dimensional representations t_2 and e respectively,

$$xy, yz, zx \qquad (t_2)$$

$$x^2 - y^2, 3z^2 - r^2 \qquad (e) \tag{3.8}$$

Symmetry considerations alone do not tell us whether the energy levels belonging to the t_2 orbitals lie lower than those

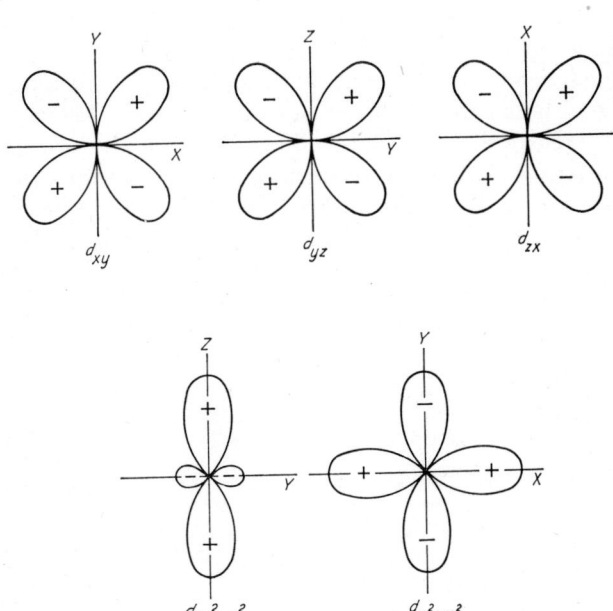

FIG. 3.2. The five d-functions showing the directions of the lobes relative to the cubic axes and also their relative signs.

belonging to the e orbitals. However, from an inspection of the form of the t_2 and e orbitals, it is expected that, for a positive ion in a tetrahedral environment, the e orbitals will have lowest energy, since their lobes are not directed towards the nearest neighbours. The converse is true for a positive ion within an octahedron of negative ions.

The electric field at an ion surrounded tetrahedrally by four nearest neighbours is given for d-states in the point charge approximation, by a potential of the form

$$V = Axyz + B(x^4 + y^4 + z^4 - 3r^4/5) \qquad (3.9)$$

Here, the first term is an odd function of the position co-ordinates and reflects the lack of inversion symmetry of the lattice site. The second term is formally identical with that for an octahedrally co-ordinated ion, but is smaller by a factor $\frac{4}{9}$. The splitting between the e and t_2 states is proportional to B.

Ludwig and Woodbury,[4,11] and Ham and Ludwig,[12] have accounted, in a qualitative way, for the observed fine structure and g-values of both substitutional and interstitial ions. The basis is a phenomenological model for the filling of the e and t_2 orbitals and is consistent with the spin resonance observations described in §3.2 (see Fig. 3.3). In this model, it is assumed that the orbitals are filled in accordance with Hund's rules, i.e. the states of both groups are singly occupied before the lowest state is doubly

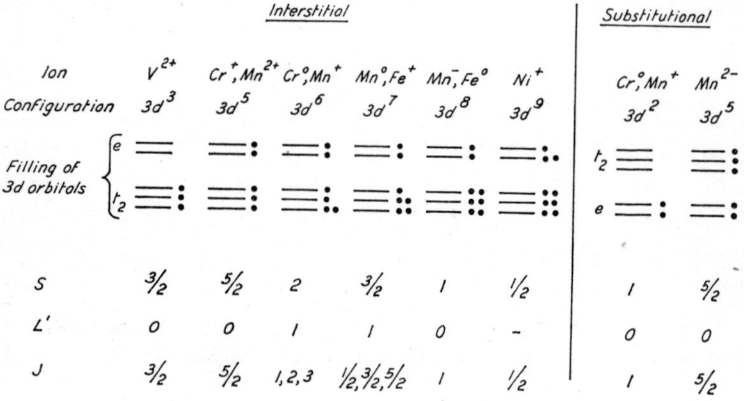

	Interstitial						Substitutional	
Ion	V^{2+}	Cr^+, Mn^{2+}	Cr^0, Mn^+	Mn^0, Fe^+	Mn^-, Fe^0	Ni^+	Cr^0, Mn^+	Mn^{2-}
Configuration	$3d^3$	$3d^5$	$3d^6$	$3d^7$	$3d^8$	$3d^9$	$3d^2$	$3d^5$
S	$3/2$	$5/2$	2	$3/2$	1	$1/2$	1	$5/2$
L'	0	0	1	1	0	$-$	0	0
J	$3/2$	$5/2$	$1,2,3$	$1/2,3/2,5/2$	1	$1/2$	1	$5/2$

Fig. 3.3. Electronic structure of transition metal ions which have been studied by electron spin resonance in silicon.
(By courtesy of G. W. Ludwig and H. H. Woodbury, and Academic Press Inc.)

occupied; the assumption is made that the energy separation between the two groups of states (usually denoted by $10D_q$) is small enough for the energy conditions to be favourable for putting an electron into an empty orbital of the upper set, with parallel spin, because of decreased Coulomb repulsion and the reduction of the energy by exchange interaction. In this connection we have just seen that D_q is only about half as large as it is for octahedral co-ordination.

The lowest terms of interest of the many-electron free ion configurations are, assuming Russell-Saunders coupling, ^2D, ^3F, ^4F, ^5D, and ^6S, and the tetrahedral crystalline field partially lifts their degeneracies in the following way:[13]

$$D \to T_2(3) + E(2)$$
$$F \to T_1(3) + T_2(3) + A_2(1) \qquad (3.10)$$
$$S \to A_1(1)$$

The numbers in parentheses indicate the dimensions of the various irreducible representations of the cubic group, i.e. the degeneracies of the resulting sets of levels (apart from spin degeneracy). For a weak field (i.e. where the crystal-field potential energy is much less than the Coulomb interactions of the electrons) the energy differences between the crystal-field levels are

$$D: \quad W(E) - W(T_2) = \pm 10D_q$$
$$F: \quad W(T_2) - W(A_2) = \tfrac{5}{4}[W(T_1) - W(T_2)] = \pm 10D_q \qquad (3.11)$$

The T_1 and T_2 states are characterized by an effective orbital angular momentum[2] $L' = 1$, and spin orbit coupling (assumed weaker than the crystal-field potential) further lifts their degeneracies.

So far no account has been taken of possible hybridization of the wave functions, nor of the effect of covalent bonding. Because of the lack of inversion symmetry of the substitutional site, hybridization of the 3d functions occurs only with those functions of the central ion having opposite parity.

Ham and Ludwig[12] neglected admixtures from states having $L > 3$ and used the following hybridized t_2 one-electron orbitals:

$$\psi_{xy} = \alpha d_{xy} + \beta p_z + \gamma f_z$$
$$\psi_{yz} = \alpha d_{yz} + \beta p_x + \gamma f_x \qquad (3.12)$$
$$\psi_{zx} = \alpha d_{zx} + \beta p_y + \gamma f_y$$

where the combinations of the various d-, p-, and f-functions are such as to give tetrahedrally directed wave functions. Hybridization of the e-states was assumed small since the lowest states with similar symmetry have $L = 5$.

According to Abragam and Pryce[2] the effective orbital angular momenta of the d-, p-, and f-states are -1, 1 and $\frac{3}{2}$ respectively. Hence there are opposite contributions to matrix elements between t-states of the orbital angular momentum, spin-orbit interaction and hyperfine interaction[12] from the d- and p-functions. These contributions are proportional to α^2 and β^2 respectively. It is expected that ions having orbitally degenerate ground states should show the effect of d-p hybridization most markedly (electron configurations $3d^3$, $3d^4$, $3d^8$, $3d^9$).

The experimental observations for substitutional ions at sites of tetrahedral symmetry show that D_q is negative and about half as large as it is for the same ions in ionic host crystals, and are in agreement with the predictions of the point ion approximation.

Covalent bonding with the ligands, via σ- or π-bonds, also changes the wave functions at the central ion. From symmetry considerations it can be seen that whereas both t_2 and e orbitals can form π-bonds with the ligands only, the t_2 orbitals can form σ-bonds.[14] Observations on particular ions in different host crystals have indicated that covalency does have a marked effect on such parameters of the E.S.R. spectrum as the g-value, the crystal-field splitting coefficient, and the hyperfine and superhyperfine interactions. For instance, for the electron configuration $3d^5$ (manganese) the magnitude of the hyperfine interaction coefficient A decreases from $97 \cdot 8 \times 10^{-4}\,\mathrm{cm}^{-1}$ for Mn^{2+} in CaF_2 (ionic)[15] to about $40 \times 10^{-4}\,\mathrm{cm}^{-1}$ for germanium and silicon.[12] Measurements of the cubic field splitting parameter a for the $^6S_{5/2}$ ground term of manganese and iron in ZnO and CdTe[16] indicate that bonding with the ligands gives a larger value than predicted by simple crystal-field theory.[17] Superhyperfine structure, which is expected to be an important feature for ions in covalently bonded lattices, has been observed for Cr^0 and Mn^+.[12]

For the ions that occupy interstitial sites the value of D_q is positive and the order of the t_2 and e states is reversed. This situation is characteristic of octahedrally co-ordinated ions. Thus it would appear that the effect of the six, octahedrally arranged, next-nearest neighbours (see Fig. 3.1) predominates over that of the four tetrahedrally arranged nearest neighbours. The ratio of the next-nearest neighbour distance to the nearest-neighbour distance is only $\frac{2}{3}$. In the phenomenological model due to Ludwig and Woodbury,[18] the spin resonance observations can be accounted for by the transfer of all valence electrons (4s) to the 3d shell, whereas for substitutional ions enough 3d electrons are transferred to the 4s shell to form tetrahedral bonds with the ligands.

We have seen in equation (3.9) that the crystalline potential contains two terms, one of which is an even function of the coordinates and the other an odd. Matrix elements of the crystalline field are of the form $\langle l'|V|l''\rangle$ where l', l'' denote the parity of the states. Remembering that both the wave functions and the potential functions can be expanded in spherical harmonics, we see that the matrix elements for the odd potential term vanish for states of definite parity. However, for hybridized wave functions in which there is admixture of states of opposite parity, as occurs for ions at sites of tetrahedral symmetry in silicon, there can be non-zero matrix elements.

Bloembergen[19,20] suggested that shifts of energy levels proportional to an applied electric field should be observable for paramagnetic ions at sites lacking inversion symmetry. If an electric field is applied, then there is an additional term $e\boldsymbol{\xi}.\mathbf{r}$ in the Hamiltonian which is an odd function of $\mathbf{r}$.

Ham[21] has considered the effect of an electric field on an ion at a site having hybridized one-electron wave functions of the following form:

$$\psi_{yz} = \alpha d_{yz} + \beta p_x + \gamma(\phi_1 - \phi_2 + \phi_3 - \phi_4)$$
$$\psi_{zx} = \quad\text{cyclic permutations} \qquad (3.13)$$
$$\psi_{xy} =$$

Here d_{yz}, etc., and p_x, etc., represent 3d and 4p orbitals on the central ion respectively, and the ϕ's are σ-orbitals from the nearest-neighbour atoms, which are combined in a way appropriate to the symmetry of the situation. The only non-zero matrix element between the states (3.13) of the perturbation $e\xi_z z$ is $\langle\psi_{yz}|e\xi_z z|\psi_{zx}\rangle$ $=p\xi_z$. Consequently, the degeneracy of these states is lifted, with $\Delta E = 0$, $\pm p\xi_z$. The parameter p can be thought of as a dipole moment. It is convenient to describe[2] this splitting by an effective angular momentum operator $\mathscr{L}'$ and

$$\mathscr{H}_\xi = -\xi_z p(\mathscr{L}_x'\mathscr{L}_y' + \mathscr{L}_y'\mathscr{L}_z') \qquad (3.14)$$

For many-electron states an effective total angular momentum $\mathbf{J} = \mathbf{L}' + \mathbf{S}$ is used and the electric field splitting is described by an operator of the form (3.14). For an applied electric field in the [001] direction, Ludwig and Ham[22] have used a spin Hamiltonian of the following form to describe the E.S.R. spectrum:

$$\mathscr{H}_\xi = \xi_z[b\beta(J_1H_1 - J_2H_2) + E(J_1^2 - J_2^2) + A_\xi(J_1I_1 - J_2I_2)$$
$$+ P_\xi(I_1^2 - I_2^2) - \gamma_\xi\beta_N(I_1H_1 - I_2H_2)] \qquad (3.15)$$

where the axes referred to by the subscripts 1, 2, 3 are the [110], [1$\bar{1}$0], and [001] directions respectively. The coefficients b, E, A_ξ, P_ξ, and γ_ξ depend on p, the spin-orbit coupling, and the energy separation between excited states.[21] When including this additional term in the total spin Hamiltonian, the spin resonance transitions between the states M_s and $M_s - 1$ are given by

$$h\nu = g\beta H + Am_I + \xi_z[b\beta H + 3E(M_s - \tfrac{1}{2})$$
$$+ A_\xi m_I]\sin^2\theta \cos 2\phi \qquad (3.16)$$

where θ and ϕ are the polar and azimuthal angles describing the direction of H ($\phi = 0$ corresponds to the [110] direction). It can be seen that there is an anisotropic shift in the electronic g-value and the hyperfine interaction, as well as a splitting of the electronic energy levels in zero magnetic field. Even where the many-electron ground state is an orbital singlet (e.g. Fe^0, Mn^-), the above effects may be observable, owing to the perturbing effect of a nearby, orbitally degenerate, excited state. For example, the ground state for Fe^0 interstitial in silicon has the electron configuration $t_2^6 e^2$ ($S = 1$, $L' = 0$). There is, however, a nearby triply degenerate excited state, corresponding to the electron configuration $t_2^5 e^3$ for which $L' = 1$, which is split by the applied electric field. Non-zero matrix elements of spin-orbit coupling, the orbital Zeeman effect and the nuclear spin-electron orbit interaction perturb the ground state, and splittings of the E.S.R. lines in an applied electric field have been observed.[23] For interstitial Cr^0

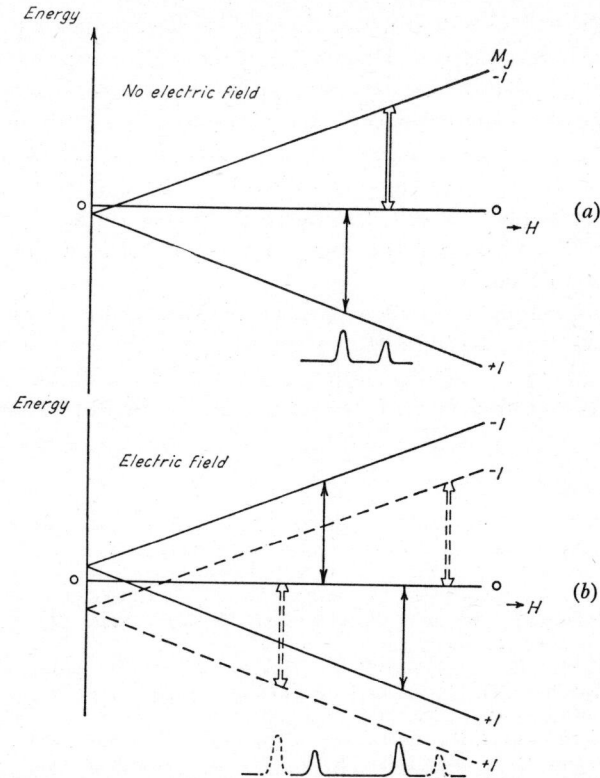

FIG. 3.4. Splitting of the spin resonance lines from interstitial Cr^0 ($J = 1$) in silicon by an applied electric field (schematic).
(a) No applied electric field; the zero field splitting is due to the perturbing effects of excited states within the $J = 2$ manifold.
(b) Electric field 10 kV/cm applied; the additional splitting in zero magnetic field is of opposite sign for interstitial sites related by the inversion operation.

($3d^6$, $J = 1$), two fine structure components are observed in zero electric field and these are shifted in opposite directions on applying an electric field.[22] As the interstitial sites fall into two classes, differing by the inversion operation, and since the effective dipole moment has opposite signs for these two sites, two pairs of lines are in fact observed (see Fig. 3.4).

The external electric field displaces the paramagnetic ion, hence a term proportional to $\xi_z xy$ is added to the crystalline-field potential.

It can be shown that externally applied electric fields and shear strains affect the spin Hamiltonian in a similar way,[22] and hence both perturbations can be described through the same parameter p.

The parameters b and E of equation (3.15) are small for ions having no orbital degeneracy and are largest for Mn^+ ($3d^6$, $S = 2, L' = 1$), having the values $8\cdot5$ ($\pm0\cdot2$)$\times 10^{-7}$ cm volt^{-1} and 25×10^{-7} cm volt^{-1} respectively. Hence for an electric field of about 10 kV cm^{-1} the energy-level splitting is of the order of $2\cdot5 \times 10^{-2}$ cm^{-1}.

Spin resonance transitions may be induced by an alternating electric field, because of the sensitivity of the energy levels to applied electric fields. Ludwig and Ham[24] have, in fact, observed electrically induced $\Delta M_s = \pm 2$ transitions for Mn^+ in silicon.

References

1. See for instance: Collins, C. B., and Carlson, R. O., *Phys. Rev.*, 1957, **108**, 1409; or Hannay, N. B., *Semiconductors*, Chapter 8 (Reinhold, 1959).
2. Abragam, A., and Pryce, M. H. L., *Proc. Roy. Soc.* 1951, **205**A, 135.
3. Low, W. *Paramagnetic Resonance in Solids* (Academic Press, 1960).
4. Ludwig, G. W., and Woodbury, H. H., *Solid State Physics*, Vol. 13 (Academic Press, 1962).
5. Bleaney, B., and Rubins, R. S., *Proc. Phys. Soc.* ,1961, **77**, 103.
6. Woodbury, H. H., and Ludwig, G. W., *Phys. Rev.*, 1960, **117**, 102.
7. Feher, G., *Phys. Rev.*, 1959, **114**, 1219.
8. Woodbury, H. H., and Ludwig, G. W., *Phys. Rev.*, 1962, **126**, 466.
9. Collins, C. B., and Carlson, R. O., *Phys. Rev.*, 1957, **108**, 1409.
10. Parasnis, A. S., and Mitchell, J. W., *Phil. Mag.*, 1959, **4**, 171.
11. Woodbury, H. H., and Ludwig, G. W., *Phys. Rev. Letters*, 1960, **5**, 96.
12. Ham, F. S., and Ludwig, G. W., *Paramagnetic Resonance*, Vol. 1, p. 130 (Academic Press, 1963).
13. Griffith, J. S., *The Theory of Transition Metal Ions*, (Cambridge University Press, 1961).
14. Coulson, C. A., *Valence*, Chapter 10 (Oxford University Press, 1961).
15. Baker, J. M., Bleaney, B., and Hayes, W., *Proc. Roy. Soc.*, 1958, **247**A, 141.
16. Hall, T. P. P., Hayes, W., and Williams, F. I. B., *Proc. Phys. Soc.*, 1961, **78**, 883.
17. Gabriel, J. R., Johnston, D. F., and Powell, M. J. D., *Proc. Roy. Soc.*, 1961, **264**A, 503.
18. Ludwig, G. W., and Woodbury, H. H., *Phys. Rev. Letters*, 1960, **5**, 98.
19. Bloembergen, N., *Science*, 1961, **133**, 1363.
20. Bloembergen, N., *Phys. Rev. Letters*, 1961, **7**, 90.
21. Ham, F. S., *Phys. Rev. Letters*, 1961, **7**, 242.
22. Ludwig, G. W. and Ham, F. S., *Paramagnetic Resonance*, Vol. 2, p. 620 (Academic Press, 1963).
23. Ludwig, G. W., and Woodbury, H. H., *Phys. Rev. Letters*, 1961, **7**, 240.
24. Ludwig, G. W., and Ham. F. S., *Phys. Rev. Letters*, 1962, **8**, 210.

Chapter 4

Radiation-Damaged Semiconductors

GENERAL FEATURES OF RADIATION DAMAGE

The effects of the bombardment of solids by high energy radiations (fast neutrons, deuterons, protons, electrons and γ-rays) have been studied* in great detail from the theoretical and practical points of view. In general, the regions of radiation damage have a very complicated structure and the interpretation of experimental observations is a difficult problem.

A minimum energy transfer to a host atom is necessary if the atom is to be permanently transferred from a lattice site to an interstitial position (Frenkel defect), and the probability of such a displacement depends on the energy of the incident particle or photon.[1] Kohn[2] has calculated that, for germanium, the threshold transfer energy for permanent displacement lies between 7 and 15 eV. The experimental values[3] for this energy have been found to lie between 14·5 and 30 eV, and are considered to be in reasonably good agreement with the theoretical estimate, bearing in mind the approximations that have to be made. In silicon and indium antimonide, the threshold energies have been found to be 12·9 eV and 5·7 eV respectively.[3]

The extent of the damage caused by a bombarding particle depends on its mass and charge. For instance, electrons and γ-rays usually produce single displaced atoms[4] (primary displacements), whereas protons and deuterons may transfer sufficient energy to the primary 'knock-on' atom to enable further displacements to occur (cascade process). For fast neutrons, much more energy is transferred to the primary knock-on atoms and the resulting cascade may involve thousands of atoms. Thus, the radiation

---

* An extensive report on radiation-damaged semiconductors can be found in *Journal of Applied Physics*, Vol. 30, 1959.

damage is contained in large clusters, whereas for electrons and
γ-rays the defects are distributed fairly uniformly and an interstitial atom remains within a few lattice spacings of its associated
vacancy.

Radical changes occur in the electrical properties of semiconductors when they are subjected to radiation by high energy
particles or photons. For instance, in n-type germanium, the
resistivity increases with radiation dose from 10^{-2} ohm cm, in a
typical sample, to about 10^2 ohm cm, after which the material
becomes p-type and the resistivity decreases to a value of about
0·1 ohm cm. This kind of behaviour is ascribed to the production
of acceptor centres during the radiation-damage process. Eventually, the acceptor centres over-compensate for the original donor
impurities, the position of the Fermi level changing appropriately.
In p-type germanium, the resistivity increases with dose and this
is attributed to an increase in scattering, which is due to the
increased number of lattice defects. The resistivities of both n- and
p-type silicon increase with radiation dose until the material
becomes virtually intrinsic at room temperature, with resistivities
in the region of 10^4 ohm cm. The explanation of this behaviour
requires the generation of both donor and acceptor centres during
the radiation-damage process.

A great deal of attention has been devoted to high energy electron
irradiation of silicon. An electron energy between about 150 and
650 keV is necessary to transfer energy equalling the threshold
energy to the primary displaced atom.[3] Easily controlled and
intense sources of electrons with energies in this range are readily
available (van der Graaf accelerators or linear accelerators). One
important advantage of using silicon is that the defects produced
are extremely stable, even at room temperature, whereas in
germanium the situation is complicated by annealing processes.
One disadvantage of using electrons is that, for energies near to
that required for transferring the threshold energy, the damage is
confined to a thin layer below the surface of the material and, in
the measurement of electrical properties, the use of very thin
samples introduces experimental difficulties.

In the interpretation of the properties of radiation-damaged
semiconductors, the principal problems arise from the complexity
of the defects, and the simultaneous existence of more than one

type of defect. The electronic energy levels of the defects have been determined by such experimental methods as measuring the rate of charge carrier removal as a function of the variation of the Fermi energy during irradiation, the temperature variation of the Hall coefficient, the effect of irradiation on the carrier lifetime and mobility,[5] the infra-red absorption,[6] and by the 'pulsed field' technique.[7] In the latter the Fermi level in a region of the semi-conductor near to the space-charge layer at the surface is forced down into the energy gap (in *n*-type material) by an applied electric field. Defect states, whose energies thus become greater than the Fermi energy, lose electrons to the conduction band by thermal excitation. Information regarding the capture cross-section and position of the defect states can be obtained by considering the kinetics of the process. An important feature of the method is that discrimination can be obtained between effects associated with surface and bulk states.

The general features of radiation-damaged semiconductors are that the principal energy levels are produced by any kind of bombardment, and that there is a large degree of symmetry between states in the upper and lower halves of the energy gap.

The experimental techniques mentioned so far are macroscopic in nature, i.e. the average effect of large numbers of effects is measured. Some information can be obtained about the microscopic structure of certain radiation-damage centres from the dichroism of the relevant infra-red absorption band when a uniaxial stress is applied.[8]

The E.S.R. technique is of great value for investigating the microscopic structure of paramagnetic defects in solids and, in particular, can yield information regarding the symmetry properties of defects. E.S.R. spectra attributed to radiation-damage centres have been observed in both *n*- and *p*-type silicon irradiated by high-energy electrons and fast neutrons. The earliest observation, by Schulz-Dubois *et al.*,[9] was in neutron-irradiated *p*-type silicon, but subsequently much more attention has been paid to electron-induced centres because of their simpler structures.

Bemski[10] and Watkins *et al.*[11] noticed that different spectra could be obtained from electron-irradiated *n*-type silicon, depending on whether the crystal was 'pulled' from a melt contained in a quartz crucible or whether it was prepared by the 'floating-zone' technique.[12] This distinction suggests that oxygen impurity atoms, which are present in comparatively high concentration (about 10^{18} atoms cm^{-3}) in pulled crystals, are an important component of the radiation-produced defect centres. In floating-zone material the oxygen content may be as low as 10^{15}–10^{16} atoms cm^{-3}.

The results of infra-red absorption experiments[13] are consistent with vibrations of an oxygen atom in a defect centre of the type proposed to explain the E.S.R. observations. Several different E.S.R. spectra have been observed and have been associated with different defect centres. They are denoted the Si–A, Si–B, Si–C, Si–E and Si–J centres.*

Important information has been obtained about the role of impurities in trapping radiation-induced primary defects and also about the mobilities of the primary defects.

§4.2

ELECTRON-IRRADIATED SILICON

Observations

The two spectra that were first investigated in detail were those attributed to the Si–A and Si–E centres. They were, after room temperature irradiation, observed in n-type silicon (N_d between 10^{15} and 10^{16} atoms cm^{-3}) at temperatures between $4 \cdot 2°$K and $20°$K. Interesting information is obtained if the intensities of the Si–A, Si–E and donor resonances are plotted as functions of electron dose for pulled and floating-zone crystals (see Fig. 4.1). In the former material the Si–A resonance grows linearly with dose and simultaneously the donor resonance decreases. As the donor resonance vanishes, the Si–A resonance begins to decrease with dose at a rate about twenty times smaller than the initial growth rate. On the other hand, in floating-zone material the Si–A resonance is extremely weak and decreases very rapidly beyond the electron

---

* In view of the large number of centres (more than 26) for which E.S.R. spectra have been observed, Watkins has proposed a new labelling scheme. For example, he suggests that the Si-A centre should be renamed Si–B1, and the Si–E centre Si–G8. The letter refers to the investigator (G stands for General Electric Research Laboratory and B for Bell Telephone Laboratory) and the numbers (1, 8, etc.) to a particular spectrum. For further details, see Watkins, G. D., *Proceedings of the Symposium on Radiation Effects in Semiconductors*, p. 97, 1964 (Dunod).

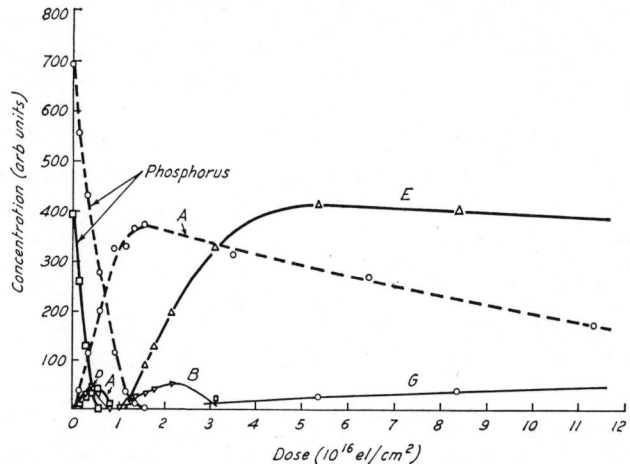

FIG. 4.1. Production of spin resonance centres in *n*-type silicon
(10^{15} phosphorus atoms cm^{-3} approximately) irradiated by 1·5 MeV
electrons at room temperature. The relative concentrations may be in
error by a factor of 1·5 to 2.
————— Floating-zone material 1·5 × 10^{15} P atoms cm^{-3}.
– – – – – 'Pulled' material 2·6 × 10^{15} P atoms cm^{-3}.
(By courtesy of G. D. Watkins *et al.*[11])

dosage (10^{16}–10^{17} electrons per cm², depending on N_d) at which
the donor resonance disappears. After further irradiation a new
resonance line, designated the Si–E resonance, appears, grows
rapidly and does not diminish significantly at large dosages.

After electron irradiation at 20°K, no Si–A resonance is observed
but it does appear, albeit with diminished intensity compared with
room temperature irradiated material, after annealing at temperatures up to 300°K.[11]

The interpretation of the dependencies of the intensities of the
various resonance lines upon electron dose in pulled crystals is as
follows. Net acceptor levels, which have been identified with a
level 0·17 eV below the conduction band,[5,13] are formed as a result
of radiation damage, and donor electrons are trapped in them.
Hence the donor resonance decreases as the Si–A resonance grows
until all the donor levels are emptied of electrons. The subsequent
slow decrease of the Si–A resonance is attributed to the formation
of a level lying 0·4 eV below the conduction band and having a

much lower production rate than the Si–A centre. The impurity responsible for the Si–A resonance must be present in concentrations significantly greater than the donor-impurity concentration used (10^{15}–10^{17} cm^{-3}) to account for the initial linear growth rate of the Si–A resonance. It must also be electrically inactive and must have a small or zero magnetic moment (absence of hyperfine interaction apart from that due to Si^{29} atoms), and this coupled with absence of the resonance in floating-zone material strongly suggested that the structure of the Si–A centre involved an oxygen atom.

In phosphorus-doped silicon, all the lines of the Si–E spectra split into two hyperfine components, probably because there is an interaction with the phosphorus impurity atom ($I = \frac{1}{2}$). The growth and decay curves of the Si–E and phosphorus resonances respectively in the irradiated floating-zone material can be explained by assuming that a net acceptor level is produced which is initially filled and non-paramagnetic. Thus the donor levels are emptied as the acceptor levels are produced and eventually the donor resonance disappears (see Fig. 4.1). The Si–E resonance appears when, as a result of the irradiation, the Fermi level moves far enough down into the energy gap for the acceptor level to lose an electron and become paramagnetic.

The annealing behaviour subsequent to low temperature irradiation strongly suggests that, in the formation of the Si–A and Si–E centres, a mobile defect is trapped at an impurity atom, i.e. the centres are not primary defects. Indeed, the annealing studies reveal that the defects (vacancies and/or interstitials) are mobile even at temperatures as low as 77°K. As we shall see, the E.S.R. results indicate that the unpaired electrons are in broken bonds suggesting that the trapped defect is a vacancy. It was these E.S.R. investigations which revealed the important role that impurities (oxygen or donor atoms) play in the formation of stable radiation-damage centres.

The decrease in the Si–A growth rate in pulled crystals with increasing phosphorus content can be accounted for by the above models for the Si–A and Si–E centres, as there would be competition for the mobile vacancies between the oxygen and phosphorus impurities.

Spin resonance spectra associated with many other defects have been observed, but only the Si–C, Si–J and Si–B centres will be discussed in detail here. The Si–B spectrum can be explained on the basis of an unpaired electron in a broken bond, but the number of vacancies associated with the defect is not known, nor has it been established whether an impurity atom is involved. The Si–C and Si–J centres are different charge states of a divacancy.

The structure of the defect centres

The E.S.R. spectra of Si–A, Si–E, Si–C, Si–J and Si–B centres can be interpreted by means of a spin Hamiltonian of the form

$$\mathcal{H} = \beta \mathbf{H} . \mathbf{g} . \mathbf{S} + \sum_j \mathbf{I}_j . \mathbf{A}_j . \mathbf{S}_j \tag{4.1}$$

where Σ_j represents a sum over neighbouring magnetic nuclei (donor-impurity nuclei or Si^{29} nuclei). The **g**- and **A**-tensors are nearly axially symmetric in all cases and, except for the **g**-tensor for the Si–C and Si–J centres, the symmetry axes are very close to the $\langle 111 \rangle$ crystalline axes. In fact, the unpaired electron in each of the centres is presumed to be in a broken bond which, in the absence of distorting effects, would point towards a vacancy (see Fig. 4.2).

The tetrahedrally-directed covalent bonds for a silicon atom at normal lattice sites are formed by sp^3 hybridization of silicon atomic wave functions. The 3s and 3p atomic wave functions are combined according to

$$\psi = p\psi_{3s} + q\psi_{3p} \tag{4.2}$$

where $q^2 = 3p^2$ and normalization requires $p^2 + q^2 = 1$. Bonding and anti-bonding wave functions between two nearest neighbour silicon atoms at the kth and lth lattice sites are of the form

$$\psi = \frac{1}{\sqrt{2}}(\psi_k + \psi_l) \tag{4.3a}$$

and

$$\psi = \frac{1}{\sqrt{2}}(\psi_k - \psi_l) \tag{4.3b}$$

respectively, and correspond to valence- and conduction-band wave functions.

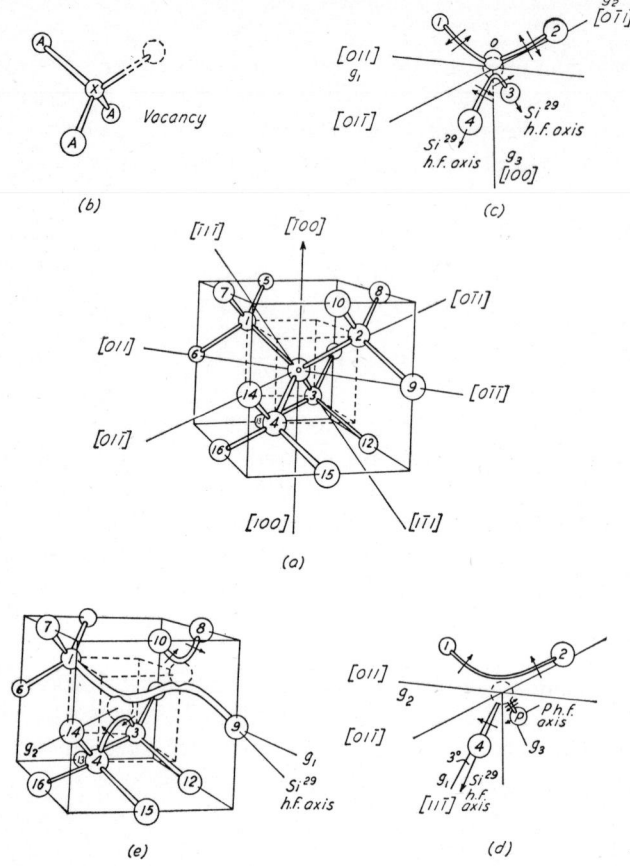

Fig. 4.2. The structures of radiation-damage centres in electron-irradiated silicon. (a) The undamaged diamond-type crystal structure. (b) Si–B centre. (c) Si–A centre. (d) Si–E centre. (e) Si–J centre.

For the unpaired electron in a broken bond the wave function can be written in the form[14]

$$\psi'(X) = \eta(\alpha\psi_{3s} + \zeta\psi_{3p}) \qquad (4.4)$$

It is expected that α and ζ will be different from p and q, owing to the asymmetry of the situation. The coefficient η represents the fact that the unpaired electron wave function will not be localized entirely on atom X but will extend over the whole defect. Thus the total wave function can be written as a linear combination of atomic orbitals (L.C.A.O.) on sites around the defect:

$$\Psi = \sum_j \eta_j \psi_j' \qquad (4.5)$$

The hyperfine interaction term in equation (4.1) includes contributions from Fermi 'contact' interactions and dipole–dipole interactions between the electron and nuclear magnetic moments. For a single electron

$$\mathcal{H}_{h.f.} = 2g_N\beta\beta_N \left[\frac{3(\mathbf{r.S})(\mathbf{r.I})}{r^5} + \frac{(1-\mathbf{S}).\mathbf{I}}{r^3} + \frac{8\pi}{3}\delta(\mathbf{r})\mathbf{S.I} \right] \quad (4.6)$$

and, when averaged over the many-electron wave function for a defect centre, can be written in the tensor form $\mathcal{H}_{h.f.} = \mathbf{I.A.S}$. The dipolar term has a $(3\cos^2\theta - 1)$ angular dependence, where θ is the angle between $\mathbf{r}$ and the axis of symmetry. Assuming, as a first approximation, that the hyperfine interaction at the jth lattice site is determined solely by the wave function ψ_j close to the site, then the hyperfine interaction is axially symmetric about the bond axis. Thus the hyperfine interaction tensor has components $\mathbf{A}_{\parallel}$, $\mathbf{A}_{\perp}$ given by

$$\mathbf{A}_{\parallel} = a + 2b \qquad (4.7a)$$

and

$$\mathbf{A}_{\perp} = a - b \qquad (4.7b)$$

where

$$a \equiv \frac{16\pi}{3} g_N\beta\beta_N\eta^2\alpha^2 |\psi_{3s}(0)_X|^2 \qquad (4.8a)$$

is the Fermi contact term and

$$b \equiv \frac{4}{5} g_N\beta\beta_N\eta^2\zeta^2 \langle r^{-3} \rangle_{3p} \qquad (4.8b)$$

is the dipolar term. The magnitudes only of $\mathbf{A}_{\parallel}$, $\mathbf{A}_{\perp}$ are determined from measurements of hyperfine splittings, but since a and b are known to be negative for Si^{29} (g_N is negative for Si^{29}), and by using tabulated Hartree functions[15,16] to calculate $|\psi_{3s}(0)_X|^2$ and $\langle r^{-3} \rangle_{3p}$, it has been possible to calculate values of $\alpha_j{}^2$, $\zeta_j{}^2$ and $\eta_j{}^2$ for equivalent silicon sites. In general, the hyperfine interactions are much larger than the line widths (2·5 gauss) and well-resolved spectra are observed.

The observed g-values show small shifts from the free electron value for all the centres. It is possible to estimate the expected g-shifts using a L.C.A.O. treatment of the simple model shown in Fig. 4.2(b). The g-shift is given by

$$\Delta g_{ij} = -2\sum \frac{\langle o|(V_{so})_i|n\rangle \langle n|L_j|o\rangle}{E_n - E_o} \qquad (4.9)$$

where

$$V_{so} = (\mathbf{E} \times \mathbf{p})\beta/mc \qquad (4.10)$$

and $\mathbf{E}$ and $\mathbf{p}$ are the electric field seen by the electron and its momentum respectively. $|o\rangle$ and $|n\rangle$ are the ground state and nth excited state of the defect centre respectively. The various contributions to Σ_n are illustrated in Fig 4.3, and the expression obtained for Δg, assuming complete localization of the unpaired electron, is[17]

$$\Delta g_\perp \simeq \zeta^2\lambda \left[\frac{1}{E_b} - \frac{1}{E_a}\right] \qquad (4.11)$$

with $\Delta g_\parallel \simeq 0$. Assuming $\lambda \sim 2 \times 10^{-2}$ eV($\frac{2}{3}$ of the atomic 3p spin-orbit coupling constant for silicon), $E_a \simeq 2\cdot5$ eV, $E_b \simeq 1\cdot5$ eV, and $\zeta^2 = 0\cdot86$, then $\Delta g_\perp \simeq 0\cdot005$. Better agreement with experimental results is obtained, than with this simple calculation, if account is taken of admixture of 1s, 2s and 2p core wave functions in the molecular wave functions. Also, owing to nuclear shielding, there is enhancement of the bonding wave functions, and a diminution of the anti-bonding wave function, near the core of an atom. Both of these effects increase the positive contribution of the g-shift and result in better agreement between the calculated and observed values.[17]

From the symmetry of the **g**-tensors and the symmetry and magnitudes of the hyperfine interactions it has been possible to obtain a detailed picture of the distribution of the unpaired electron wave function in the defect centres.

Because of the delocalized nature of the wave functions of the unpaired electron ($\eta^2 < 1$), it is expected that there will be a small negative contribution to Δg, since spin resonance experiments on delocalized electrons and holes (see §§2.2 and 2.8) have revealed negative g-shifts. Such contributions in fact cause the total g-shift to be negative for certain of the components of the **g**-tensors in the Si–E, Si–C, and Si–J centres.

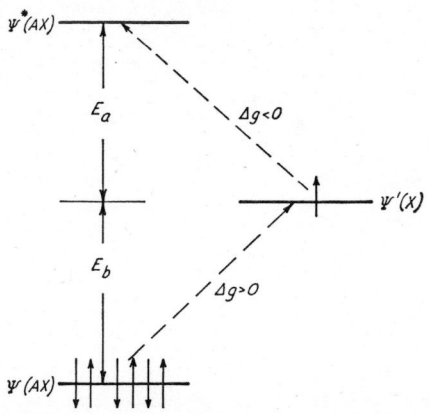

FIG. 4.3. Electron states for an atom next to a vacancy. $\psi(AX)$ and $\psi^*(AX)$ are the bonding and anti-bonding orbitals between atoms A and X respectively (see Fig. 4.2b), and $\psi'(X)$ is the broken bond orbital. The transitions used in calculating the g-shift are shown.
(By courtesy of G. D. Watkins and J. W. Corbett.[17])

For the Si–B centre the **g**-tensor is almost axially symmetric around a bond direction $[\bar{1}\bar{1}1]$ with a very small g-shift in this direction. The large hyperfine interaction with one Si^{29} nucleus is also axially symmetric and this leads to the model of an unpaired electron in a broken bond pointing almost directly towards a vacant lattice site. An analysis of the hyperfine interaction reveals enhanced p-character in the wave function of the unpaired electron (86 per cent p-character). This is compatible with a pulling of the atom X [see Fig. 4.2(b)] away from the vacancy with a resulting tendency to form planar sp^2 orbitals with its three nearest neighbours, leaving the broken bond with enhanced p-character.

In the Si–A spin resonance spectrum the axes of the hyperfine interaction with Si^{29} atoms lie very close to the $[11\bar{1}]$ and $[1\bar{1}1]$ crystallographic axes. No O^{17} hyperfine structure was observed

TABLE 4.1 Results for radiation-damage centres in silicon, showing the s and p character of the orbital in which the unpaired electron is predominately located*

Centre	Position	g	α^2 (s)	ζ^2 (p)	η^2	Percentage of total electron wave function involved
			Wave function coefficients			
Si–B	About $E_g/2$	$g_1 = 2\cdot0026 \pm 0\cdot0003$ $g_2 = 2\cdot0085 \pm 0\cdot0003$ $g_3 = 2\cdot0107 \pm 0\cdot0003$	0·14	0·86	0·64	64
Si–A	$E_c - 0\cdot17$ eV	$g_1 = 2\cdot0092 \pm 0\cdot0003$ $g_2 = 2\cdot0026 \pm 0\cdot0003$ $g_3 = 2\cdot0033 \pm 0\cdot0003$	0·37	0·63	0·36 on each of 1 and 2	72
Si–E	$E_c - 0\cdot4$ eV approx.	$g_1 = 2\cdot0005 \pm 0\cdot0003$ $g_2 = 2\cdot0112 \pm 0\cdot0003$ $g_3 = 2\cdot0096 \pm 0\cdot0003$	0·19	0·81	0·59	59
Si–C	About $E_g/2$	$g_1 = 2\cdot0012 \pm 0\cdot0003$ $g_2 = 2\cdot0135 \pm 0\cdot0003$ $g_3 = 2\cdot0150 \pm 0\cdot0003$	0·22	0·78	0·28	56
Si–J	$E_v + 0\cdot27$ eV (?)		0·16	0·84	0·31	62

* The results are taken from Watkins et al.[14]

even in samples which contained oxygen enriched to approximately
1·5 per cent O^{17}. The model for the Si–A centre[15] is shown in
Fig. 4.2(c), and, in the neutral state, all of the Si–O and Si–Si bonds
contain two paired-off electrons. The additional trapped electron
goes into an anti-bonding orbital between silicon atoms at sites
3 and 4. As the oxygen atom lies at a node of this anti-bonding
orbital, the absence of O^{17} hyperfine interaction is consistent with
this model. From the Si^{29} hyperfine interaction measurements it
was calculated that 71 per cent of the unpaired electron wave
function is associated with the anti-bonding wave functions on
atoms 3 and 4, and the remainder is spread over between 12 and 16
neighbouring sites. For the Si–Si anti-bonding wave function,
there is enhanced s-character (37 per cent—see Table 4.1), which
indicates that atoms 3 and 4 are pulled in towards the vacancy. The
presence of oxygen has been confirmed by infra-red absorption
experiments in electron-irradiated silicon.[8]

The spin resonance spectrum of the Si–E spectrum in phosphorus-doped silicon shows an intense central group of lines, each
of which is split into a doublet, together with satellite lines with
an intensity 20 times smaller, which also show doublet structure.
The interpretation of this spectrum is that the satellite lines are
due to strong hyperfine interaction with one Si^{29} nucleus (4·7 per
cent abundant) and that the doublet splitting is due to hyperfine
interaction with a phosphorus atom associated with the centre.[14,17]
E.N.D.O.R. measurements[17] enabled the magnetic moment of the
nucleus causing the doublet splitting to be measured and confirmed
that it was phosphorus. From an analysis of the **g**-tensor anisotropy
and the hyperfine interactions Watkins and Corbett proposed for
the Si–E centre the model shown in Fig. 4.2(d), in which a vacancy
is trapped next to a substitutional phosphorus atom. Two of the
silicon atoms surrounding the vacancy pair off, leaving broken
bonds on one silicon atom and on the phosphorus atom. There are
two electrons available for the broken bond on the latter, as it is a
Group V atom, and these pair off, leaving an unpaired electron in
the broken bond on the remaining silicon atom. This accounts for
the large hyperfine interaction with one Si^{29} atom and for the
centre being paramagnetic when neutral.

In Watkins and Corbett's model the degeneracy of the broken
bond orbitals on the three silicon atoms lying nearest to the vacancy

is removed by a Jahn–Teller distortion,[18] as shown in Fig. 4.4. The measurements of the hyperfine interactions show that the unpaired electron is 60 per cent localized in the broken bond orbital. Of the remaining portion of the wave function 3 per cent is accounted for on each of the silicon atoms 1 and 2, and 1 per cent on the phosphorus atom. That portion of the unpaired electron

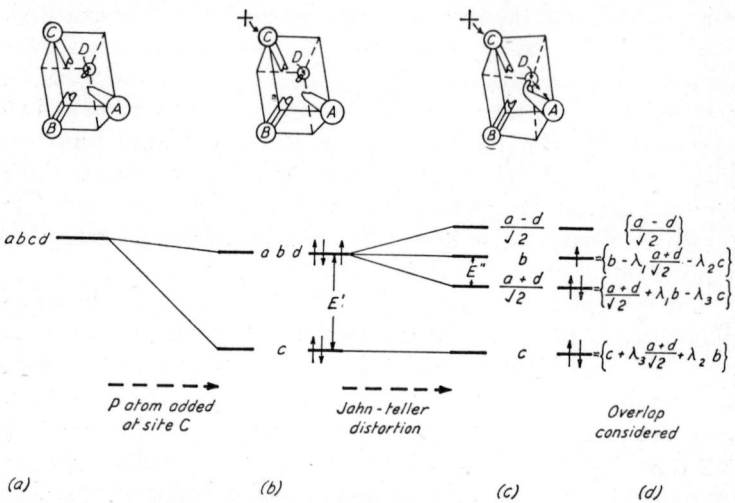

Fig. 4.4. Simple L.C.A.O. molecular orbital model of the electronic structure of the E-centre.

(a) Four degenerate (ignoring overlap) orbitals of the isolated vacancy.

(b) The lowering of the c orbital due to the extra nuclear charge of the phosphorus atom at C.

(c) Lifting of the degeneracy of the a, b, d orbitals by a Jahn–Teller distortion.

(d) Modifications to the wave functions when small overlap between the atomic orbitals is considered. (These wave functions are orthogonal and normalized only through first order in the λ_i.)

(By courtesy of G. D. Watkins and J. W. Corbett.[17])

wave function on atom 4 has 86 per cent p-character and this represents a 'pulling-away' of the atom from the vacancy by its three nearest neighbours. The 33 per cent of the wave function unaccounted for is assumed to be distributed over more distant neighbours of the vacancy and gives rise to unresolved, or at best partially resolved, hyperfine structure.

Two spin resonance spectra whose intensity depended on the energy of the bombarding electrons were observed by Bemski *et al.*,[19] and by Corbett and Watkins.[20] The spectra appeared after irradiation at 20°K, where vacancies and interstitials are not mobile, which suggested that the associated centres were primary defects. Also, the spectra were not observed for electron energies ≤ 0·5 MeV, indicating that a threshold energy was necessary for their production. Increasingly complex defects are produced for higher bombarding energies, owing to secondary displacements,[1] and it seemed possible that the centres consisted of divacancies. This interpretation has been supported by the determination of the axes of the **g**-tensor and Si^{29} hyperfine interaction [see Fig. 4.2(*e*)], and by studies of thermally- and stress-induced alignments of differently orientated equivalent divacancies.[20]

The Si–J resonance is observed in *p*-type material and the Si–C resonance in high resistivity *n*-type material, corresponding to the broken bond containing one or three electrons respectively (one in an anti-bonding broken bond orbital). It appears that the bond can accept a fourth electron since the resonance is not observed in low resistivity *n*-type material.

An interesting observation by Corbett and Watkins was that the production rate for the divacancies was dependent on the direction of the electron beam relative to the crystal axes of the specimen. For a particular beam energy, the maximum energy imparted to the primary recoil atom (which in turn displaces a second atom) occurs when the recoil is in the beam direction. Hence, as the beam energy is reduced, most divacancies will be produced if the electron beam is in a ⟨111⟩ direction. By monitoring the relative intensities of the components of the resonance spectrum due to divacancies lying in equivalent ⟨111⟩ directions, the anticipated anisotropy of divacancy production was observed.

A general feature of the models for defect centres which have been presented, is the existence of equivalent structures which may arise in two ways. Firstly, at temperatures in the region of 150°K or higher, the whole defect may seek energetically preferred equivalent orientations in the lattice in strained crystals. By observing the recovery of the intensities of the components of the spin resonance spectrum corresponding to differently oriented defects, after the stress has been removed, it is possible to estimate

the potential barrier that has to be overcome in the thermally
activated re-orientation process. Secondly, there may be a redistribution of the oxygen atom in the Si–A centre, or of the
unpaired electron in the Si–E centre, between the silicon atoms
surrounding the vacancy, i.e. there is electronic redistribution.

For the Si–E centre at temperatures below $100°K$, where
re-orientation does not occur, thermally-activated electronic redistribution has been observed through lifetime broadening and
motional narrowing effects. The lifetime τ_l of the states corresponding to the various electronic distributions can be determined
by measuring the width $\Delta\omega$ at half-height of the resonance line,
where the line shape is given by

$$g(\omega) = \{[1 + (\omega_0 - \omega)^2/(\Delta\omega)^2]\pi\Delta\omega\}^{-1} \qquad (4.12)$$

and

$$\Delta\omega = 1/T_2 \qquad (4.13)$$

(see pp. 33 to 34). The relationship between T_2 and τ_l has been
determined by Gutowsky and Saika[21] for the extreme cases where
the redistribution causes (*a*) broadening and (*b*) motional narrowing of the observed spectrum. Corbett and Watkins[17] found that
they could fit their results to

$$(\tau_l)^{-1} = 1 \cdot 6 \times 10^{12} \exp(-E/kT) \qquad (4.14)$$

with $E = (6 \cdot 22 \pm 0 \cdot 15) \times 10^{-2}$ eV. Measurements of the Si^{29} hyperfine interaction revealed a three-fold increase in the intensity of
the satellite lines, owing to hyperfine interaction with Si^{29} atoms
at the 1 and 2 sites, and a reduction of the splitting to 51 gauss.
This can be attributed to an increased spreading of the unpaired
electron wave function over the two sites, with a corresponding
increase in the probability of finding a Si^{29} at one of the sites, and
to a reduction of the strength of the hyperfine interaction. This
evidence clearly indicates that it is not a molecular re-orientation
that occurs, but rather an electron redistribution in which the
unpaired electron is in a molecular orbital extending over all the
sites associated with the defect.

The electronic redistributions have been analysed in terms of
Boltzmann factors which characterize the populations of the
energy levels corresponding to defects with different orientations

relative to an applied uniaxial stress. Consider the Si–A centre. For a $\langle 110 \rangle$ stress there are three non-equivalent orientations and hence two Boltzmann factors are required. On the other hand, for a $\langle 100 \rangle$ or a $\langle 111 \rangle$ stress, only one Boltzmann factor is required, since there are only two non-equivalent directions. Corbett and Watkins[15,17] assumed that the change in energy of the defect was due primarily to alteration of the Si–Si distance [between atoms 3 and 4 of Fig. 4.2(*c*)]. In this situation and for a $[01\bar{1}]$ stress

$$\frac{n_{12}}{n_{34}} = \exp(-T_\alpha/T)$$

$$\frac{n_{12}}{n_{13}} = \exp(-T_\beta/T)$$

(4.15)

where 12 indicates the defect with the unpaired electron trapped in the anti-bonding orbital between silicon atoms at sites 1 and 2, the populations of the other three possible orientations being equal to n_{13}. Boltzmann population distributions characterized by T_γ and T_δ can be obtained in a similar way for stresses in $\langle 100 \rangle$ and $\langle 111 \rangle$ directions. Values for T_α, etc., have been determined from measurements of the amplitudes of the components of the spin resonance spectrum, corresponding to defects orientated in the relevant directions, and indicate that the greatest energy change occurs for defects in which the Si–Si bond is most compressed by the applied stress (defect 34 in the notation of Fig. 4.2). Also, from the observation that T_α is negative, it is apparent that the energy of the defect is raised when these two silicon atoms are pushed together, which confirms the earlier assumption that the trapped electron is in an anti-bonding orbital.

The measurements of the analogous Boltzmann factors for Si–E centres indicate that the energy of the defect is lowered most when the stress is in such a direction that silicon atoms 1 and 2 [see Fig. 4.2(*d*)] are pushed together, as would be expected on the basis of covalent bonding.

The stresses used in these experiments have been in the range 12 000 p.s.i. to 26 000 p.s.i.

It has also been possible to deduce extremely useful information concerning the activation energies for re-alignment and diffusion of defects from observations on the relaxation of the spin resonance

7

spectra after removal of the stress. The silicon samples are stressed at elevated temperatures (120–145°K for Si–A centres and room temperature for Si–E centres) and the recovery monitored at 20·4°K for Si–E centres.

By fitting the time characterizing the recovery of the spin resonance spectrum to expressions of the form of equation (4.14), the activation energies for re-orientation for the Si–A, Si–E, Si–J and Si–C centres can be found. For the Si–A and Si–E centres these energies are 0·38 and 0·93 eV respectively. Care has to be taken in interpreting these activation energies in terms of the models for the defects. Consider, for instance, the case of initially *n*-type material in which the concentration of Si–A centres is ten times greater than the donor impurity concentration. The electronic redistribution time is given by

$$(\tau_{el})^{-1} = 5 \times 10^{13} \exp(-E/kT) \qquad (4.16)$$

and the time characterizing re-orientation is given by

$$(\tau_{ro})^{-1} = 3 \times 10^{12} \exp(-E/kT) \qquad (4.17)$$

Thus, at the temperatures at which the re-orientation experiments were carried out (in the region of 120–145°K), τ_{ro}/τ_{el} is about $17 . e^{20}$ and an electron can be redistributed many times during τ_{ro}. Hence, as a Si–A centre will have a trapped electron for only 10 per cent of the time, the experiments really measure the properties of neutral Si–A centres. The probable re-orientation mechanism is a rotation about one Si–O bond after the breaking of the other.

In Si–E centres, interesting information concerning the diffusion of phosphorus-vacancy pairs is obtained from a detailed consideration of the most probable re-orientation process.[17] Referring to Figs. 4.2(a) and 4.2(d), this consists of the vacancy hopping from site o to site 12 via sites 4 and 15, and the site linked to sites 9, 15 and 12. (N.B. Interchange of the vacancy and the phosphorus atom does not cause a re-orientation of the defect). The phosphorus-vacancy separation is greatest when the vacancy is at site 15, the 'next-next-nearest neighbour' site. It is supposed that the activation energy is larger than that for isolated vacancy diffusion (0·33 eV), because the defect must partially dissociate during the process. The combination of this re-orientation process and the interchange of the phosphorus atom and the vacancy is in effect a translation, or diffusion, of the whole defect.

From the decay rate for the Si–E spectrum at room temperature in unstrained material, Corbett and Watkins estimated a time constant $\gtrsim 4 \times 10^6$ sec, whereas the defect is re-orientating once every 400 sec, i.e. the vacancy escapes and the defect dissociates only once in about 10^4 opportunities, giving a barrier against dissociation ~ 0.25 eV. This is in rough agreement with the Coulomb interaction energy (0.28 eV) for a single positive charge and a single negative charge, which are separated from each other by the next-next-nearest neighbour distance in a medium having a dielectric constant of 12, thus providing additional support for the model.

There is, because of this binding energy, a greater probability of finding a vacancy near a phosphorus atom than near a silicon atom. By adding this to the measured activation energy of 3.66 eV for phosphorus diffusion,[22] Corbett and Watkins estimate an activation energy of 3.94 eV for silicon self-diffusion. This result is of great interest as this important quantity has not been measured directly.

In the Si–C and Si–J centres, both electronic redistribution and re-orientation can occur with activation energies ~ 0.06 eV and ~ 1.3 eV respectively. Referring to Fig. 4.2(*e*), we see that the extended bond containing the unpaired electron could also connect atoms 10 and 3, or 8 and 4, and the electronic redistribution occurs between these equivalent situations.

§4.3

NEUTRON-IRRADIATED SILICON

It is expected that the defects produced by neutron irradiation will be more complex than for electron irradiation, since it has been estimated that each primary knock-on atom produces about 200 secondary displacements.[23]

The resonance spectra are complex[9,24] and depend on the position of the Fermi level and on annealing processes. Nisenoff and Fan[25] made detailed studies on heavily irradiated (i.e. near intrinsic) silicon. Two advantages of working with such material are its high resistivity, which allows measurements to be made above room temperature, and the negligible shift of the Fermi level during annealing processes. From the intensity of the spin resonance spectrum it was concluded that, although the concentration of paramagnetic defects was proportional to the neutron dose, the production rate was 200 times smaller than the estimated number of displaced atoms (20 per neutron–cm). The spectra, whose g-values were in the region of 2·0, were independent of the type of doping and also of the method of growth (floating-zone or pulled).

Nisenoff and Fan[25] carried out annealing experiments to simplify the spin resonance spectrum and designated the most intense portion of the spectrum which remained, the Si–N centre. The **g**-tensor and Si^{29} hyperfine structure both have almost axial symmetry about the $\langle 111 \rangle$ directions and the simplest defect that would fit this evidence, is an isolated vacancy. However, evidence was presented in connection with the Si–A centre which showed that the isolated vacancies (Si–B centres) are mobile below room temperature, whereas the Si–N spectrum required annealing at temperatures of 440°K, or higher, for its production. Hence, it was concluded that the Si–N and Si–B centres were not one and the same defect.

References

1. Seitz, F., and Koehler, J. S., *Solid State Physics*, Vol. 2, p. 331 (Academic Press, 1956).
2. Kohn, W., *Phys. Rev.*, 1954, **94**, A1409.
3. Loferski, J. J., and Rappaport, P., *J. Appl. Phys.*, 1959, **30**, 1296.
4. Cahn, J. H., *J. Appl. Phys.*, 1959, **30**, 1310.
5. Wertheim, G. K., *Phys. Rev.*, 1958, **110**, 1272.
6. Fan, H. Y., and Ramdas, A. K., *J. Appl. Phys.*, 1959, **30**, 1127.
7. Rupprecht, G., and Klein, C. A., *Phys. Rev.*, 1959, **116**, 342.
8. Corbett, J. W., Watkins, G. D., Chrenko, R. M., and McDonald, R. S., *Phys. Rev.*, 1961, **121**, 1015.
9. Schulz-Dubois, E., Nisenoff, M., Fan, H. Y., and Lark-Horovitz, K., *Phys. Rev.*, 1955, **98**, 1561.
10. Bemski, G., *J. Appl. Phys.*, 1959, **30**, 1195.
11. Watkins, G. D., Corbett, J. W., and Walker, R. M., *J. Appl. Phys.*, 1959, **30**, 1198.
12. Hannay, N. B., (Ed.) *Semiconductors*, Chapter 3 (Reinhold, 1959).
13. Hill, D. E., Thesis, Purdue University (1959, unpublished).
14. Watkins, G. D., and Corbett, J. W., *Disc. Faraday Soc.*, 1961, **31**, 86.
15. Watkins, G. D., and Corbett, J. W., *Phys. Rev.*, 1961, **121**, 1001.
16. Hartree, W., Hartree, D. R., and Manning M. F., *Phys. Rev.*, 1941, **60**, 857.
17. Watkins, G. D., and Corbett, J. W., *Phys. Rev.*, 1964, **134**, A1359.

18. Jahn, H. A., and Teller, E., *Proc. Roy. Soc.* 1939, **161**A, 220.
19. Bemski, G., Szymanski, B., and Wright, K., *J. Phys. Chem. Solids*, 1963, **24**, 1.
20. Corbett, J. W., and Watkins, G. D., *Phys. Rev. Letters*, 1961, **7**, 314.
21. Gutowsky, H. S., and Saika, A., *J. Chem. Phys.*, 1953, **21**, 1688.
22. Watkins, G. D., *J. Phys. Soc. Japan*, 1963, **18** (Suppl. 2), 22.
23. Lark-Horovitz, K., *Semiconducting Materials*, p. 47 (Academic Press, 1951).
24. Nisenoff, M., and Fan, H. Y., *Bull. Am. Phys. Soc.*, 1959, **4**, 159.
25. Nisenoff, M., and Fan, H. Y., *Phys. Rev.*, 1962. **128**, 1605.

Chapter 5

Electron Spin Resonance
in Germanium
and Group III–V Compounds

For a number of fundamental reasons, which will be considered later in this chapter, and also because of technological difficulties, there have been far fewer E.S.R. observations for germanium and the Group III–V compounds than for silicon. The technological difficulties, which arise with the Group III–V compounds, concern the production of single crystals, which must be sufficiently pure to prevent effects due to accidental impurities masking or seriously modifying those due to deliberately introduced impurities.

§5.1

GERMANIUM

Although large, highly purified, single crystals of germanium were available before single crystals of silicon of similar purity, the former material has not been such a fruitful field for E.S.R. experiments. There are three fundamental reasons for this. Firstly, the spin-orbit interaction for the valence band is about an order of magnitude larger for germanium than for silicon, resulting in much shorter spin-lattice relaxation times. Secondly, the ground state of shallow donor impurities is very sensitive to strain. Hence, random local strains in the crystal produce a spread of g-values, which are incompletely averaged out by motional narrowing,[1] thus causing an increase in the line width. Thirdly, the donor-electron wave function is more 'peaked' around the donor-impurity nucleus for germanium than for silicon. This means that unresolved hyperfine interaction with 7·77 per cent abundant Ge^{73} $(I = \frac{9}{2})$ causes a greater line width than does the interaction with 4·7 per cent abundant Si^{29} in n-type silicon.

As the dielectric constant of germanium is higher than that of silicon, the 'radii' of the donor-impurity centres are greater than those in silicon (see §1.3). Thus, in germanium, the donor electrons become delocalized for the smaller values of N_d through the overlap of the wave functions of neighbouring donor centres. Whereas in silicon significant overlap occurs for $N_d \sim 5 \times 10^{17}$ cm^{-3}, in germanium the corresponding concentration is $\sim 5 \times 10^{16}$ cm^{-3}.

Following studies of excitons[2] which revealed a g-value for conduction electrons of 1·6, Feher *et al.*[3] observed E.S.R. at liquid helium temperatures, both from electrons bound to shallow donor impurities and from non-localized electrons. The g-values in unstressed samples of phosphorus- and arsenic-doped material were 1·5631 ± 0·0003 and 1·5701 ± 0·0003 respectively. The values of $g_\parallel$ and $g_\perp$ for electrons moving in a single valley have been found from experiments on stressed crystals[4,5] analogous to those described for silicon in §2.3, and the results are shown in Table 5.1.

Roth[6] has calculated the g-values for conduction electrons in semiconductors on a two-band model and this is expected to be more applicable to germanium than to silicon. The reason for this is that the spin-orbit splitting of the valence band is not required to vanish at the zone boundary in the direction where the conduction-band minimum occurs, and hence the dominant contribution to the g-shift comes from the valence band. In silicon we saw that the dominant contribution to the g-shift came from the deep-lying 2p core states.[7] The expressions obtained by Roth for $g_\parallel$ and $g_\perp$ are

$$g_\parallel = 2 - \frac{\delta}{E_{13'}}\left(\frac{m_e}{m_\perp} - 1\right) \tag{5.1a}$$

and

$$g_\perp = 2 - \frac{\delta}{E_{13'}}\left(\frac{m_e}{m_\parallel} - 1\right) \tag{5.1b}$$

Here, $E_{13'}$ is the energy gap between the valence band and the conduction band at the zone boundary in a $\langle 111 \rangle$ direction, and δ is the spin-orbit splitting of the valence band at that point. Taking $\delta = 0 \cdot 18$ eV and $E_{13'} = 2 \cdot 1$ eV[8] and using $m_\parallel/m_e = 1 \cdot 60$ and $m_\perp/m_e = 0 \cdot 08$, the calculated values for $g_\parallel$ and $g_\perp$ are 0·98 and 2·07 respectively. The agreement with the experimental values is quite good for $g_\parallel$, but the observed shift of $g_\perp$ from the free electron value is opposite to that predicted by Roth's theory. As $\delta g_\perp$ is quite small, it is thought that contributions to the g-shift from bands other than the valence band may be significant.

From the observation of resolved hyperfine structure it was concluded that, of the singlet and triplet states into which the effective-mass-theory ground state is split, the singlet state lies lowest. For this state, in which all four valleys contribute equally to the wave function, the g-value is isotropic, being given by

$$g_0 = \tfrac{1}{3}g_\parallel + \tfrac{2}{3}g_\perp \qquad (5.2)$$

Thus the calculated value for g_0 is 1·71.

For low enough donor-impurity concentrations, resolved hyperfine spectra consisting of $2I + 1$ lines, where I is the spin quantum number of the donor-impurity nucleus, have been observed in phosphorus-, arsenic-, and bismuth-doped germanium. The unresolved structure due to hyperfine interaction with Ge^{73} nuclei will be considered later. Measurements of the resolved hyperfine structure yield, of course, values of $|\Psi(0)|^2$ for the donor-electron wave function, the form of which we must consider. According to the effective mass theory, the ground state is four-fold degenerate with

$$\Psi^i(\mathbf{r}) = \sum_{j=1}^{4} \alpha_j F_j(\mathbf{r}) u_j(\mathbf{r}) \exp(i\mathbf{k}_j . \mathbf{r}) \qquad (i = 1 \ldots 4) \qquad (5.3)$$

Because of the breakdown of the effective mass theory near the donor-impurity nucleus, the degeneracy is partially lifted, resulting in a singly—and a triply—degenerate state given by

$$\alpha_j^1 = \frac{1}{2}(1, 1, 1, 1) \qquad \text{singlet} \qquad (5.4a)$$

and

$$\left. \begin{aligned} \alpha_j^2 &= \frac{1}{2}(1, \quad 1, -1, -1) \\[4pt] \alpha_j^3 &= \frac{1}{\sqrt{2}}(1, -1, \quad 0, \quad 0) \\[4pt] \alpha_j^4 &= \frac{1}{\sqrt{2}}(0, \quad 0, \quad 1, -1) \end{aligned} \right\} \quad \text{triplet} \qquad (5.4b)$$

As $|\Psi(0)|^2$ is large for the singlet and vanishes for the triplet, the existence of well-resolved hyperfine structure indicates that the singlet is the ground state. In fact, for the singlet, the theory yields

$$|\Psi(0)|^2 = 4|F(0)|^2.|u(\mathbf{r}_l)|^2 \qquad (5\cdot5)$$

where $|u(\mathbf{r}_l)|^2$ is the probability density of a conduction-band Bloch function at a lattice site, the Bloch function being normalized so that

$$\frac{1}{\Omega} \int_{\text{cell}} |u(\mathbf{r})|^2 \, d\mathbf{r} = 1$$

where Ω is the volume of the unit cell.

As the donor wave functions are less compressed in germanium than in silicon, one would expect that the hyperfine interaction to be smaller since $|F(0)|^2$ is smaller. However, in fact the observed hyperfine splittings are of the same order of magnitude as those in silicon (see Table 5.1). This is attributed to the previously-mentioned 'peaking' of the donor wave function at the donor nucleus, i.e. to an enhanced value of $|u(\mathbf{r}_l)|^2$ in equation (5.5). From measurements on Si^{29} nuclei of the relaxation rate due to the fluctuating 'contact' hyperfine interaction with conduction electrons[9,10]

$$\frac{|u(\mathbf{r}_l)|^2_{Si}}{\langle |u(\mathbf{r})|^2 \rangle_{Av\ Si}}$$

was measured to be 178, where the average is taken over a unit cell. Wilson [5] used a measured value for the relaxation time of Ge^{73} nuclei obtained by Wyluda[11] to calculate a value for $|u(\mathbf{r}_l)|^2_{Ge}/|u(\mathbf{r}_l)|^2_{Si}$ of 9·5 and hence obtained $|u(\mathbf{r}_l)|^2_{Ge} = 1700 \pm 300$, since $\langle |u(\mathbf{r})|^2 \rangle_{Av\ over\ cell} = 1$. On substituting this quantity into equation (5.5) and using the value of $|F(0)|^2$ obtained from effective mass theory,[12] the calculated value for the hyperfine splitting is about an order of magnitude smaller than the observed splittings. The central-cell correction to $F(\mathbf{r})$ (see §1.3) increases $|F(0)|^2$ by almost an order of magnitude and this brings the calculated hyperfine splitting into reasonable agreement with that observed.

The valley-orbit splitting E_{13} between the singlet and triplet states has been obtained from measurements of the hyperfine splitting as a function of uniaxial strain. For a uniaxial compressive

TABLE 5.1 Results on shallow donor centres in germanium

Donor Impurity	Optical ionization energy (eV)	g_0	$g_{\parallel}$	$g_{\perp}$	(ΔH) Ge^{73} (gauss)	Total h.f.s. (gauss)	$\lvert\Psi(o)\rvert^2$ ($\times 10^{24}$ cm^{-3})	Valley-orbit splitting E_{13} (eV)	Wave funtion spread a_0^* (Å) Expt.	Theory	Energy of triplet state below conduction band (eV)
Phosphorus	0·0125	1·5631 ±0·0002	0·83 ±0·05	1·93 ±0·02	10±1	21±1	0·17	0·0029	31·8	38·5	0·0096
Arsenic	0·0145	1·5700 ±0·0002	0·87 ±0·04	1·92 ±0·02	11±1	107±3	0·69	0·0042	29·8	36·8	0·0103
Bismuth	0·0123	1·5671 ±0·0004			10±1	944±5	2·15	0·0028	31·8	39·0	0·0095
Antimony	0·0098							0·00057			0·0093
Theoretical value		1·70	0·98	2·07							0·0092

stress in a $\langle 110 \rangle$ direction, the two conduction-band minima lying in the plane containing the stress axis are lowered in energy and the other two minima are raised in energy. Wilson[5] has calculated the resulting amount of admixture of the triplet state into the ground state and, assuming that the only effect of the stress is to cause a redistribution of the populations of the minima, the hyperfine splitting is given by

$$\frac{(h.f.s.)_{\text{strain}}}{(h.f.s.)_0} = \tfrac{1}{2}[1 + (1 + x^2/9)^{-1/2}] \qquad (5.6)$$

where $x = D_u S/E_{13}$, and D_u and S are the deformation potential and applied strain respectively.

In the limit of a large $\langle 110 \rangle$ stress the hyperfine splitting would be one-half of its original value and for a $\langle 111 \rangle$ stress, in which the three minima not on the stress axis are raised in energy, the limiting value of the splitting would be $(h.f.s.)_0/4$ in the limit of large stresses.

Values have been obtained for D_u/E_{13} by fitting the observed hyperfine splittings in stressed samples to equation (5.6). For the range of strains used (up to 0.55×10^{-3}) there was a linear dependence of x on applied strain, thus confirming the validity of the assumption concerning the repopulation of the minima. Experiments by Fritzsche[13,14,15] on the effect of uniaxial stress on transport properties, such as impurity conduction and piezo-resistance in n-type germanium, yielded values for E_{13}/D_u in good agreement with Wilson's values and gave for D_u a value of 19.2 ± 0.4 eV at $6.6°$K. By using this value for D_u, the values for E_{13} shown in Table 5.1 were obtained, and by subtracting these from the optical ionization energies of the donor centres,[16] the positions of the triplet levels E_3, relative to the conduction-band edge, can be calculated for the various shallow donor impurities. All the triplet levels lie close to the value 0.0092 eV predicted by the effective mass theory, the surprising feature being that E_{13} has the same value for bismuth and phosphorus since, as we have seen, $|\Psi(0)|^2$ differs considerably for these two impurities.

The widths of the components of the E.S.R. spectra are highly anisotropic, having a minimum value when the magnetic field is directed along a $\langle 100 \rangle$ direction. In this orientation the widths are in the region of 10 gauss and about five times greater than those in silicon.

If the magnetic field is directed along a $\langle 100 \rangle$ direction, then g-shifts due to strains vanish. The reason for this is that all the minima are equivalent with respect to this direction and hence differences in the populations of the different minima are irrelevant. For orientations off the $\langle 100 \rangle$ directions, random strains in the crystal cause a spread of g-values and hence a broadening of the resonance line. Wilson[5] estimated the line width due to random strains for small angles θ between the magnetic field and the [100] axis by assuming a Gaussian strain distribution with an average component ΔS in an arbitrary $\langle 111 \rangle$ direction, and obtained

$$(\Delta H)^2 = \left(\frac{\Delta g}{g_0} \cdot H\right)^2 \tag{5.7}$$

where

$$\Delta g = \frac{(g_{\parallel} - g_{\perp})}{3g_0} \cdot \frac{2D_u \Delta S}{9E_{13}} \cdot (\sin^2\theta + \sqrt{2} \sin 2\theta) \tag{5.8}$$

In silicon, this mechanism does not produce an observable line broadening, or anisotropy of line width, since $(g_{\parallel} - g_0)$ is three orders of magnitude smaller.

Measurements of line broadening versus θ have been correlated with dislocation densities (obtained by etch pit counting) and the line widths have been found to be greatly increased in plastically deformed samples. Further evidence in favour of the notion of line broadening due to random strains has been obtained from crystals doped by neutron bombardment by means of the reaction

$$\text{Ge}^{74} + n \rightarrow \text{As}^{75} \tag{5.9}$$

The important feature of this method of doping is that the resulting donor impurities are distributed randomly throughout the crystal and are not associated with edge dislocations, as probably are the donor impurities introduced during the growth process. Thus, in the latter type of material, the average strain at the donor-impurity sites will be high and the line width will be correspondingly increased.

Further evidence concerning the clustering of donor impurities around edge dislocations has been furnished by measurements of the width of the motionally narrowed line which appears for $N_d >$ 10^{15} cm^{-3} approximately. For high enough donor-impurity concentrations, there is a probability of electrons hopping from one donor to another, because of the overlap of the donor wave functions. In this case the donor hyperfine interaction is averaged out and a single motionally narrowed line appears. From the theory of Anderson and Weiss[1] the width of such a line is given by

$$\Delta H = \frac{g\beta}{h} \frac{\Delta H^2_{h.f.s.}}{w} \tag{5.10}$$

where $\Delta H_{h.f.s.}$ is the hyperfine splitting and w is the average hopping frequency. Miller and Abraham[17] have considered the impurity band-conduction process that arises from this electron-hopping process and find for the hopping rate the expression

$$w = \left(\frac{1}{57\pi^{1/2}}\right)\left(\frac{D_u}{\epsilon}\right)^2 \cdot \frac{1}{\rho_0 c^5 a^{*2}} \cdot \left(\frac{R}{a^*}\right)^{3/2} \cdot \exp\left(-\frac{2R}{a^*}\right) \cdot E_h$$

$$\times \coth\left(\frac{\Delta}{2kT} + 1\right) \tag{5.11}$$

Here R is the average donor-impurity separation ($0.62\,N_d^{1/3}$), a^* an effective radius of the donor state (see later), and E_h the activation energy for hopping. By substituting for w in (5.10) from (5.11) and comparing the resultant equation with measurements of line width versus average donor separation, Wilson[5] found $a^* = 260$ Å and 100 Å for phosphorus and arsenic respectively. The corresponding values obtained from the effective mass theory are 70 Å and 60 Å respectively. The discrepancies suggest that the donor impurities are clustered to a certain extent and not randomly arranged. This clustering probably occurs around dislocations. From the variation of line width with temperature the activation energies for the hopping process were estimated to be 3.5×10^{-4} eV and 5.5×10^{-4} eV for arsenic and phosphorus respectively. As the g-values for the various donor impurities are different, and equal to the values for isolated impurities, it is concluded that the electrons spend most of their time at the donor sites.

The residual line width at the [100] orientation in lightly doped samples, which is due to unresolved hyperfine interaction with Ge^{73} nuclei, can be calculated, as for silicon, by assuming a random distribution of these nuclei around a donor-impurity site and is given by

$$\Delta H_{Ge^{73}} = \frac{32\pi}{g} \cdot \frac{\mu_{Ge}}{I_{Ge}} (\bar{m}_l)_{r.m.s.} \cdot \frac{f^{1/2}\eta}{4} \cdot \sum_l n_l |\exp[i\mathbf{k}_j.\mathbf{r}_l.F_j(\mathbf{r}_l)]|^4$$

$$(5.12)$$

Here μ_{Ge} and I_{Ge} are the nuclear magnetic moment and nuclear spin quantum number of Ge^{73}, m_l is the magnetic quantum number for the Ge^{73} nucleus, f is the fractional abundance of Ge^{73} nuclei, and the sum is over successive shells of lattice sites (n_l is the number of lattice sites in each shell). In order to evaluate an expression of this type for Si^{29} in silicon, Kohn[18] introduced an approximation for the non-spherical function $F(\mathbf{r})$ in which an effective radius a^* is used, where $a^* = (a^2 b)^{1/3}$ (see equation 1.18). Further, the value of a^* was derived from the observed donor ionization energy using the expression

$$a_0^* = \left(\frac{E_{eff. \ mass \ theory}}{E_{observed}} \right)^{1/2} a^*$$

$$(5.13)$$

The resultant expression for $\Delta H_{Ge^{73}}$ is

$$\Delta H_{Ge^{73}} = \frac{36}{3g} \cdot \frac{\mu_{Ge}}{I_{Ge}} (\bar{m}_l)_{r.m.s.} f^{1/2} \cdot \eta \cdot \frac{1}{(a_l a_0^*)^{3/2}} \qquad (5.14)$$

where a_l is the lattice constant. Thus we see that measurements of line width yield information concerning the extent of the donor wave functions (see Table 5.1.) The observed line widths vary little from donor to donor and this suggests that the spread of the donor wave function is so large that differences which exist near the donor nucleus affect the line width to only a small extent.

The measurement of relaxation times in germanium is made difficult by their small values (in the region of 10^{-3} sec at $1\cdot2°K$) and also by the poor signal-to-noise ratio which precludes the use of adiabatic fast passage techniques. Thus the power-saturation technique has been used,[19,5] but the results are estimated to be accurate to only about 40 per cent, because of difficulties of analysis for a situation in which $w_m T_s \simeq 1$, where $w_m/2\pi$ is the field modulation frequency employed (e.g. $w_m/2\pi = 100$ c/s, $T_s = 10^{-3}$ sec). By using an isotopically enriched sample,* Wilson reduced the line width due to hyperfine interaction with Ge^{73} nuclei by a factor of three, and thus increased the signal-to-noise ratio correspondingly.

From the measurements of variation of relaxation time with temperature, magnetic field and crystal orientation, it is clear that a T_s rather than a T_x relaxation process is dominant (see Fig. 6.3). In fact, the results (see Fig. 5.1) are in good agreement with the theories of Roth[20] and Hasegawa[21] which give for a relaxation process arising from modulation of the **g**-tensor by phonons (one-phonon process) the following expression for $(T_s)^{-1}$:

$$(T_s)^{-1} = \frac{4}{\pi}\left(\frac{g_\| - g_\perp}{g_0}\right)^2 \cdot \left(\frac{D_u}{E_{13}}\right) \cdot \frac{1}{\rho_0 u^5}\left(\frac{g\beta H}{\hbar}\right)^4 \cdot kT . f(\theta, \phi)$$

$$(5.15)$$

Here ρ_0 is the density of germanium, u is the velocity of sound and the angular function has the values 1, $\frac{1}{2}$, and $\frac{1}{3}$ in germanium for the magnetic field in the $\langle 100 \rangle$, $\langle 110 \rangle$, and $\langle 111 \rangle$ directions respectively. At temperatures where two-phonon (Raman) processes become probable, Roth and Hasegawa suggest a quadratic magnetic field dependence and a T^7 temperature dependence. In Fig. 5.1. the transition to a T^7 dependence is clearly indicated and measurements at X and K band are consistent with a H^4 dependence in the one-phonon region.

Although antimony is a shallow donor impurity, the observed spin resonance spectra differ in character from those observed in phosphorus-, arsenic-, and bismuth-doped germanium. The donor wave function is less compressed for antimony centres (ionization energy 0·0098 eV) and hence the donor electrons become delocalized at lower donor-impurity concentrations than for the other shallow donor impurities. In addition, the valley-orbit

*	Ge^{70}	Ge^{72}	Ge^{73}	Ge^{74}	Ge^{75}
			(percentage)		
Normal Germanium	20·5	27·4	7·8	36·6	7·8
Enriched Germanium	0·8	1	0·9	96·8	0·6

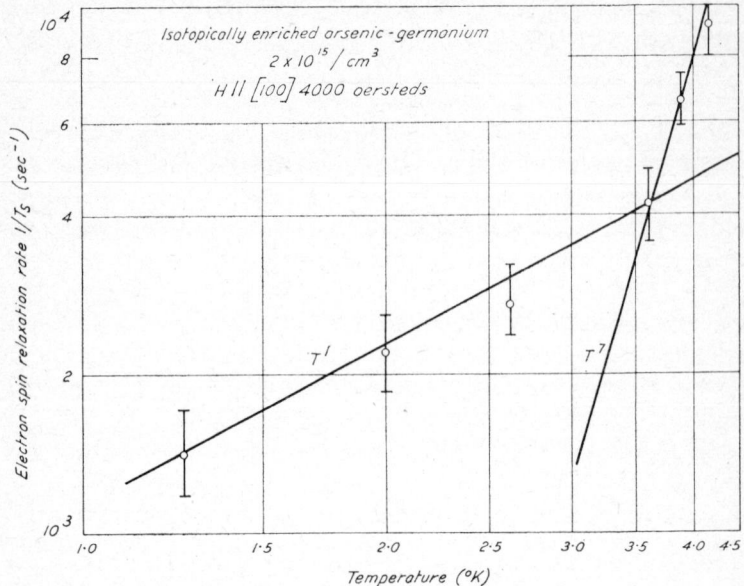

FIG. 5.1. The temperature dependence of the spin-lattice relaxation time for electrons bound to phosphorus atoms in germanium.
(By courtesy of D. K. Wilson.[5])

splitting is very small for antimony ($0\cdot00057$ eV)[22] and this means that built-in strains can cause significant changes in the ground-state wave function. Taking D_u as 19 eV and using $D_u S_c \sim E_{13}$, then the critical strain S_c is $\sim 3 \times 10^{-5}$. Strains of this magnitude are commonly found in pulled crystals of germanium and hence the nature of the spectrum observed depends strongly on the specimen used.

In addition to the single motionally narrowed line observed by Feher *et al.*,[3] and Wilson[5] ($g_0 = 1\cdot6$ in [100] direction), Pontinen and Sanders[23] observed a four-line spectrum, which reduced to three lines when the large magnetic field was in a $\{110\}$ plane and could be fitted to a spheroidal **g**-tensor of the form

$$g^2 = g_{\parallel}{}^2 \cos^2\phi + g_{\perp}{}^2 \sin^2\phi$$

The spectrum reduces to three lines for the above orientation of the large magnetic field, since the symmetry axes of two of the **g**-tensors lie in the (110) plane and the other two lie out of the plane but making equal angles with it.

Keyes and Price[24] have interpreted the observations in antimony-doped germanium by dividing the donors into three classes: (*a*) those subject to a strain with a component greater than S_c in a $\langle 111 \rangle$ direction, (*b*) those in an area where the strain is negligible and (*c*) other antimony atoms. Donors of class (*c*) will have a continuous distribution of *g*-values and hence will not give rise to an observable line, whilst those in class (*b*) give rise to the motionally narrowed single line spectrum. This model explains the fact that the intensity of the class (*a*) resonance arises from only a small fraction ($\frac{1}{40}$ approximately) of the donor impurity atoms and also the absence of this resonance in arsenic-doped germanium. In the latter material, E_{13} is about an order of magnitude larger than it is for antimony, and hence S_c will be attained over a smaller volume of the specimen. There is a much weaker temperature dependence of the intensity of class (*a*) resonance compared with class (*b*). In the latter case the separation of the ground state from the first excited state (the triplet state) is quite small, while for the class (*a*) centres, whose ground-state wave function consists of a strong admixture of triplet and singlet wave functions, the separation to the first excited state will be relatively large.

E.S.R. has also been observed for the transition metals manganese and nickel, which, as in silicon, give deep impurity levels. It is thought that both of these impurities occupy substitutional sites and accept enough electrons to complete the tetrahedral bonding.[25]

The manganese spectrum is characterized by $J = S = \frac{5}{2}$ and $g \simeq 2$ and the impurity is thought to enter the lattice as Mn^{2-}. A feature of the spectrum is that the hyperfine interaction with Mn^{55} is small compared with the value in ionic crystals. This may be due to core polarization effects or to covalency.

For nickel Ludwig and Woodbury[26] have suggested that the nickel is displaced in a $\langle 100 \rangle$ direction from a substitutional site with the principal axes of the spectrum in the [100] direction and in two mutually perpendicular directions. Another suggestion which they have made is that the nickel ion forms bonds with only two of its four nearest neighbours.

8

§5.2

GROUP III–V COMPOUNDS

E.S.R. has so far only been observed in indium antimonide, indium arsenide, gallium arsenide and gallium phosphide. The presence of residual impurities and the difficulty of controlled doping have hindered work in this field.

Delocalized electrons

Because the electron effective masses are very small (in the range $0 \cdot 013 \, m_e$ to $0 \cdot 07 \, m_e$), the radii of the shallow donor-impurity states are very large (80 Å to 640 Å). Hence, even with the minimum level of impurity concentration at present available, the donor wave functions overlap, impurity bands are formed, and the donor electrons are delocalized.

In indium antimonide the conduction band has a minimum at the centre of the first Brillouin zone and is very nearly parabolic in this region.[27] The band structure of gallium arsenide has been calculated from that of germanium by perturbation methods (gallium and arsenic lie on either side of germanium in the system of elements) and is similar in form, but with the minimum of the conduction band occurring at the centre of the zone.[27] Magneto-resistance and piezo-resistance measurements are consistent with such a 'spherical' band edge (equi-energy surfaces are approximately spherical).

The minimum energy gap is very small ($0 \cdot 18$ eV) and occurs at the centre of the zone; this simplifies the calculation of the g-value of the conduction electrons, for which Roth *et al.*[28] used a two-band model and found

$$g = 2 - \frac{2\delta}{(3E_g + 2\delta)}\left(\frac{m_e}{m^*} - 1\right) \qquad (5.16)$$

Here δ is the spin-orbit splitting of the valence band, E_g is the energy gap at $k = 0$ and m^* is the electron effective mass. Using $E_g = 0 \cdot 18$ eV, $\delta = 0 \cdot 9$ eV[29] and $m_e/m^* = 77$, equation (5.16) gives $g \simeq -56$.

Bemski[30] observed a resonance line from conduction electrons at $1 \cdot 2°$K and $4 \cdot 2°$K in samples of n-type indium antimonide containing between 2×10^{14} electrons cm^{-3} and 3×10^{15} electrons cm^{-3}, the line being superimposed on a much broader plasma resonance line.

By making observations at both 9 kMc/s and 24 kMc/s, it was verified that the additional line was not due to a plasma resonance or to cyclotron resonance. The magnitude of the measured g-value varied from 50·7 to 48·8, depending on the concentration of conduction electrons and being smallest for the highest concentration of electrons. All the samples used were degenerate at liquid helium temperatures and, therefore, only electrons in the highest Landau level contributed to the spin resonance signal. The change in g-value with increasing electron concentration is attributed to a departure of the conduction band from a parabolic form, i.e. to an increase in effective mass as the energy of the highest filled band increases. The width of the line increased from 2 gauss for a sample having 2×10^{14} electrons cm^{-3} to 23 gauss for a sample having 3×10^{15} electrons cm^{-3}. No E.S.R. was observed in samples having 10^{16} electrons cm^{-3}, presumably owing to the increase in line width with concentration.

Duncan and Schneider[31] have observed two E.S.R. lines in single crystals of n-type gallium arsenide at 4·2°K. The early experiments, made at 4·2°K and at 300 Mc/s, revealed an asymmetric line, and further experiments at 600 Mc/s and 8825 Mc/s resolved this into two distinct lines. One line ($g = 0·52$) was approximately ten times more intense than the other ($g = 1·2$). The g-value was also calculated by using equation (5.16), and the values obtained agreed with the experimental values for the more intense line to within about 10 per cent. As with indium antimonide, a variation of g-value was observed corresponding to a change in energy of the highest occupied level in specimens of different electron concentration. It was concluded that the line at $g = 0·52$ was due to delocalized electrons, probably moving in an impurity band.

Localized impurity centres

E.S.R. spectra attributed to manganese, iron, and nickel and to heat-treatment centres have been observed in gallium arsenide, gallium phosphide, and indium arsenide. The results are particularly interesting inasmuch as they give further information regarding the effects of covalency on E.S.R. spectra, and can be

TABLE 5.2 Experimental results for localized centres in Group III — V compounds

Impurity	Number of reference	Temp. (°K)	g	δg	Cubic field splitting parameter a ($\times 10^4$ cm^{-1})	Line width ΔH (gauss)	Hyperfine interaction constant A (gauss)
Iron in gallium arsenide	32	1·3	2·0462 ∓0·0006	+0·044	+339·7±0·3	54±2	10 approx.
	32	77	2·0453 ±0·0008	+0·043	+342·2±0·5		
	36	77	2·0424 ±0·0004	+0·040	+330±2		
	33	77	2·05	+0·05	+330 approx.	51·6	
Iron in indium arsenide	42	1·3	2·035 ±0·0002	+0·033	+421±1	125±3 [100] 132±3 [111]	
Iron in gallium phosphide	37	10	2·025	+0·023	+390		
Manganese in gallium arsenide	34	77	2·004	+0·002	3·3	56 approx.	56 approx.
Nickel in gallium arsenide	36	1·3	2·106 ±0·008	+0·104			

compared with the spectra for the same ions in Group IV semi-conductors, Group II–VI compounds and ionic crystals.

The spectra of manganese in gallium arsenide and iron in gallium arsenide, indium arsenide and gallium phosphide are characterized by $J = S = \frac{5}{2}$, i.e. the impurity atoms form S-state ions. This suggests that iron ($3d^6 4s^2$) substitutes for gallium or indium, as the case may be, forming a neutral centre with one 3d electron being promoted to the valence shell to take part in the covalent bonding. Similarly, manganese ($3d^5 4s^2$) is thought to form an acceptor with the two 4s electrons, partially satisfying the requirements of tetrahedrally coordinated covalent bonds. The observed g-shifts are large and positive, the zero field splitting is larger than in ionic compounds, and there is a large hyperfine interaction with neighbouring nuclei of the host crystal which may or may not be resolved.

The spin sextuplet is split by the cubic field into a quadruplet and a doublet, and the spin Hamiltonian is conveniently written in the form

$$\mathscr{H} = g\beta \mathbf{S}.\mathbf{H} + \frac{a}{6}\left[S_\xi^4 + S_\eta^4 + S_\zeta^4 - \frac{S}{5}(S+1)(3S^2 + 3S - 1) \right]$$

$$(5.17)$$

where 3a is the zero-field splitting between the doublet and quadruplet states and ξ, η, ζ are the cubic crystalline axes.

In iron-doped gallium arsenide the five fine structure lines due to $\Delta m_s = \pm 1$ transitions are well resolved and, in addition, nine of the ten possible forbidden transitions with $|\Delta m_s| > 1$ have been observed.[32] There are some discrepancies between the values of a and g obtained by different workers (see Table 5.2). De Wit and Estle[32] found a close correlation between the iron content of their crystals and the intensity of the observed E.S.R. spectrum. In contrast, Goldstein and Almeleh[33] found little correlation between the intensity of the spectrum in heat-treated gallium arsenide and the iron content as determined by mass spectrometry and, although the spectrum had many of the features common to iron, attributed it to lattice defects.

The observed spectrum in manganese-doped gallium arsenide consists of six lines, for which the g-value and position of the individual components are independent of the orientation of the

magnetic field in the (110) plane. Almeleh and Goldstein[34] assume
that the six lines are hyperfine components due to the nuclear spin
of Mn^{55} ($I = \frac{5}{2}$). The width of the hyperfine lines, which was

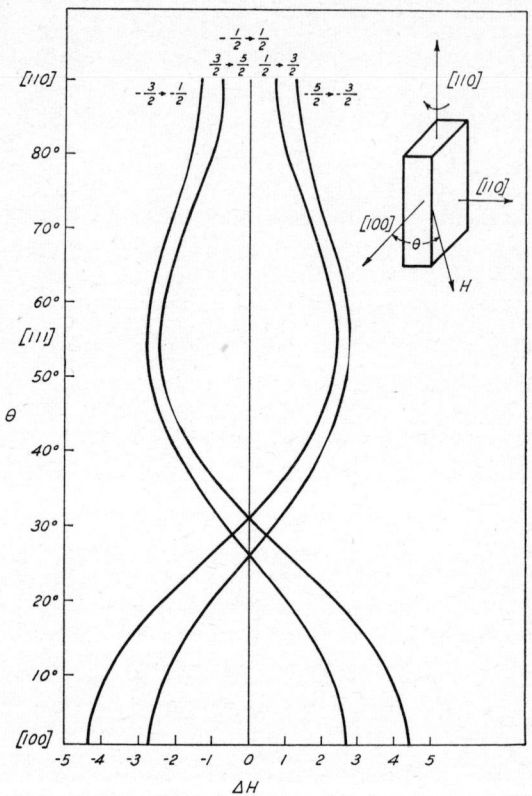

Fig. 5.2. The predicted angular dependence of the fine structure
transitions for manganese in gallium arsenide as a function of the
angle between the magnetic field and the [100] axis.
(By courtesy of N. Almeleh and B. Goldstein.[34])

anisotropic and rather large (about 56 gauss), was independent of
temperature between 77°K and 4°K, indicating that there was no
lifetime broadening of the lines by relaxation effects. The anisotropy of the line width was explained by assuming that the hyperfine lines were the envelopes of the fine structure pattern (five lines).
Matarrese and Kikuchi[35] have calculated the frequencies of the

fine structure transitions in terms of the angle θ between the magnetic field and the [100] axis. It can be seen from Fig. 5.2 that the hyperfine lines should be best resolved for that value of θ for which the separation of the fine structure lines is at a minimum.

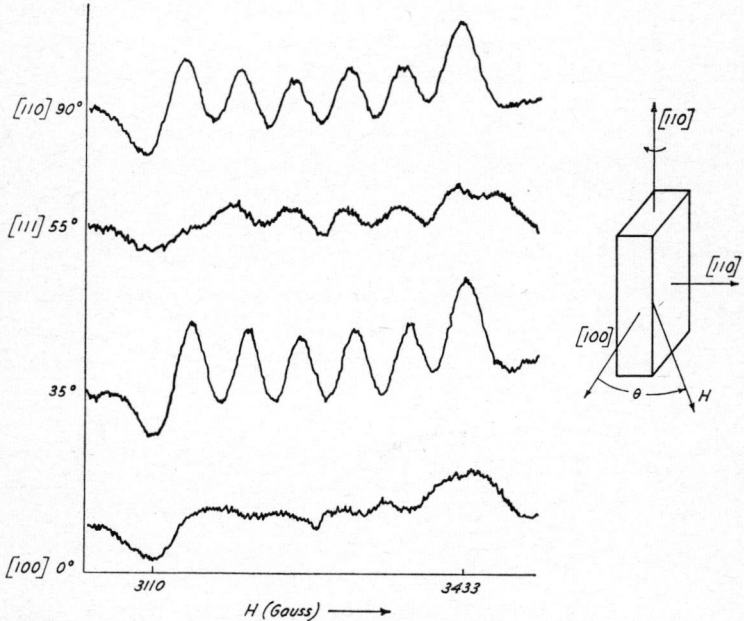

FIG. 5.3. The E.S.R. spectrum of manganese in gallium arsenide showing the variation in resolution of the hyperfine lines.
(By courtesy of N. Almeleh and B. Goldstein.[34])

Fairly close agreement was found with this prediction (see Fig. 5.3). Additional confirmation of this interpretation is given by the fact that the observed E.S.R. spectrum is independent of angle for the magnetic field rotated in the (111) plane for which θ is constant. From their measurements, Almeleh and Goldstein placed an upper limit of $3 \cdot 28 \times 10^{-4} \, \mathrm{cm}^{-1}$ on the cubic field splitting parameter a. The width of the fine structure components was estimated to be about 20 gauss and is probably due to unresolved hyperfine interaction with the nearest neighbour arsenic ($I = \frac{3}{2}$) and gallium ($I = \frac{3}{2}$) atoms.

In nickel-doped gallium arsenide, a single isotropic E.S.R. line has been observed with $g = 2 \cdot 106 \pm 0 \cdot 008$ and a width of 130 gauss.[36] Woodbury and Ludwig[37] have observed a line in manganese-doped gallium phosphide but, although it was presumed that again $J = S = \frac{5}{2}$, only the $m_s = +\frac{1}{2}$ to $m_s = -\frac{1}{2}$ transition was seen. It was suggested that the other transitions were broadened beyond detection by crystalline strains.

Considerable attention is being paid to the theoretical interpretation of E.S.R. spectra in covalently bonded compounds. Fidone and Stevens,[38] and Watanabe[39] have pointed out that, in calculating g-shifts, account must be taken of charge transfer states in which electrons may be transferred between the impurity and near neighbour host-atoms. Such a transfer leads to a positive g-shift which may be several times larger than the shift due to the excited states of the ion itself. This effect can also contribute to the zero field splitting parameter a.

An interesting feature of the spectra of iron in gallium arsenide and indium arsenide is that the ratio of the line widths (due to unresolved hyperfine interactions) is approximately equal to the weighted means of the isotopes of gallium and indium.[40] Now the nearest gallium and indium atoms to a substitutional iron atom lie at next-nearest neighbour sites, and assuming that the hyperfine interaction occurs at these sites, then the delocalization of the 3d electrons is the same in both compounds. This conclusion is consistent with results obtained for manganese in Group II–VI compounds.

Shallow acceptor-impurity centres in gallium arsenide

The investigation of the properties and mode of operation of semiconductor lasers has increased the interest in the structure of the energy bands and impurity centres of the Group III–V compounds, particularly in gallium arsenide.

Cadmium and zinc (Group II atoms) form shallow acceptor centres in gallium arsenide with ionization energies $\sim 0 \cdot 05$ eV, and their wave functions can be considered as linear combinations of the wave functions for holes in the valence band.

As in silicon, a large uniaxial stress is applied to remove the degeneracy of the acceptor levels, enabling the acceptor resonance to be observed. Title[41] observed a resonance with $g_\perp = 8 \cdot 1 \pm 0 \cdot 1$ in zinc-doped material (3×10^{17} zinc atoms cm^{-3}) with a stress of $1 \cdot 8$ kg cm^{-2} applied in the [100] direction. The g-value for cadmium centres (5×10^{16} cadmium atoms cm^{-3}) was observed to be $6 \cdot 7 \pm 0 \cdot 1$. This smaller value was expected for the more tightly bound (higher ionization energy) cadmium centres. For free holes, Luttinger[42] estimated that $g = 4K$, where K is the anti-symmetric constant for the valence band. For germanium, to which gallium arsenide is expected to be similar, Kohn[18] has estimated that K has the value $3 \cdot 5 \pm 0 \cdot 2$. From his results Title estimated $K > 2 \cdot 0$, which is in rough agreement with Kohn's value.

References

1. Anderson, P. W., Weiss, P. R., *Rev. mod. Phys.*, 1953, **25**, 269.
2. Button, K. J., Roth, L. M., Kleiner, W. H., Zwerdling, S., Lax, B., *Phys. Rev. Letters*, 1959, **2**, 161.
3. Feher, G., Wilson, D. K., and Gere, E. A., *Phys. Rev. Letters*, 1959, **3**, 25.
4. Morigaki, K., and Mitsuma, T., *J. Phys. Soc. Japan*, 1963, **18**, 462.
5. Wilson, D. K., *Phys. Rev.*, 1964, **134**, A265.
6. Roth, L. M., *Phys. Rev.*, 1960, **118**, 1534.
7. Liu, L., *Phys. Rev.*, 1962, **126**, 1317.
8. Tauc, J., and Antoncik, E., *Phys. Rev. Letters*, 1960, **5**, 253.
9. Shulman, R., and Wyluda, B., *Phys. Rev.*, 1956, **103**, 1127.
10. Lampel, G., and Solomon, I., *C. R. Acad. Sci.*, 1964, **258**, 2289.
11. Wyluda, B., *J. Phys. Chem. Solids*, 1962, **23**, 63.
12. Kohn, W., and Luttinger, J. M., *Phys. Rev.*, 1955, **97**, 1721.
13. Fritzsche, H., *Phys. Rev.*, 1959, **115**, 336.
14. Fritzsche, H., *Phys. Rev.*, 1962, **125**, 1552.
15. Fritzsche, H., *Phys. Rev.*, 1962, **125**, 1560.
16. Fan, H. Y., and Fisher, P., *J. Phys. Chem. Solids*, 1962, **8**, 270.
17. Miller, A., and Abraham, E., *Phys. Rev.*, 1960, **120**, 745.
18. Kohn, W., *Solid State Physics*, Vol. 5 (Academic Press, 1957).
19. Bloembergen, N., Purcell, E. M., and Pound, R. V., *Phys. Rev.*, 1948, **73**, 679.
20. Roth, L. M., *Phys. Rev.*, 1960, **118**, 1534.
21. Hasegawa, H., *Phys. Rev.*, 1960, **118**, 1523.
22. Fritzsche, H., *Phys. Rev.*, 1960, **120**, 1120.
23. Pontinen, R. E., and Sanders, T. M., *Phys. Rev. Letters*, 1960, **5**, 311.
24. Keyes, R. W., and Price, P. J., *Phys. Rev. Letters*, 1960, **5**, 473.
25. Hannay, N. B., *Semiconductors*, p. 340 (Reinhold, 1959).
26. Ludwig, G. W., and Woodbury, H. H., *Solid State Physics*, Vol. 13, (Academic Press, 1962).
27. Hilsum, C., and Rose-Innes, A. C., *Semiconducting III–V Compounds*, (Pergamon, 1961).
28. Roth, L. M., Lax, B., and Zwerdling, S., *Phys. Rev.*, 1959, **114**, 90.
29. Kane, E. O., *J. Phys. Chem. Solids*, 1957, **1**, 249.
30. Bemski, G., *Phys. Rev. Letters*, 1960, **4**, 62.

31. Duncan, W., and Schneider, E. E., *Phys. Rev. Letters*, 1963, **7**, 23.
32. De Wit, M., and Estle, T. L., *Phys. Rev.*, 1963, **132**, 195.
33. Goldstein, B., and Almeleh, N., *Appl. Phys. Letters*, 1963, **2**, 130.
34. Almeleh, N., and Goldstein, B., *Phys. Rev.*, 1962, **128**, 1568.
35. Matarrese, M., and Kikuchi, C., *J. Phys. Chem. Solids*, 1956, **1**, 117.
36. Bleekrode, R., Dielman, J., and Vegter, H. J., *Philips Research Reports*, 1962, **17**, 513.
37. Woodbury, H. H., and Ludwig, G. W., *Bull. Amer. Phys. Soc.*, 1961, **6**, 118.
38. Fidone, I., and Stevens, K. W. H., *Proc. Phys. Soc.*, 1959, **73**, 116.
39. Watanabe, H., *Bull. Amer. Phys. Soc.*, 1963, **8**, 439.
40. Estle, T. L., *Phys. Rev.*, 1964, **136**, A1702.
41. Title, R. S., *I.B.M. Journal*, 1963 (January), 68.
42. Luttinger, J. M., *Phys. Rev.*, 1955, **102**, 1030.

Chapter 6

Application of Electron Spin Resonance in Semiconductors

§6.1

ELECTRON TRANSFER PROCESSES IN SILICON

The E.S.R. technique has been used in a number of experiments to monitor the transfer of electrons from donor centres to acceptor centres, to measure electron-hole recombination times, to investigate electron interchange between donor centres and the conduction band, and to obtain information about impurity conduction processes.

Consider a sample of silicon containing N_d donor-impurity centres and N_a acceptor-impurity centres. If $N_d > N_a$, then, at low temperatures, there will be N_d^+ ionized donor impurities, where $N_d^+ = N_a$. If $N_d < N_a$, then all the donor impurities will be ionized, their electrons having been trapped at N_d of the acceptor impurities (see Fig. 6.1). By illuminating samples with radiation for which $h\nu > E_g$ (so-called 'intrinsic' radiation), electron-hole pairs can be created through inter-band transitions, and if extrinsic radiation, for which $E_g > h\nu > E_d$ (where E_d is the donor ionization energy), is used, then donor electrons can be delocalized.

Bemski and Szymanski[1] investigated samples of p-type silicon (boron-doped) that contained compensating donor impurities. No E.S.R. was observed initially, since all the donor impurities were ionized, but after illumination with intrinsic radiation (wavelength of 1·03 micron) the E.S.R. spectra, characteristic of the donor impurity, were observed. The intensity of the spectrum depended on the photon flux up to a saturation value and did not decay over

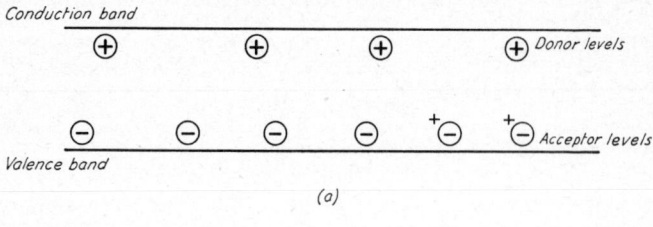

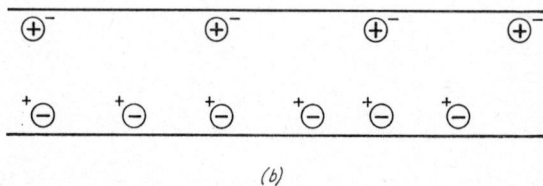

Fig. 6.1. The distribution of electrons amongst the donor and acceptor impurities in silicon ($N_d < N_a$) (a) under dark conditions and (b) after illumination with intrinsic radiation. In (b) the free electrons generated by the radiation have been trapped at the previously positively ionized donor impurities.

a period of hours after cutting off the illumination. It was assumed that the free electrons were trapped at the ionized donor centres. From Hall effect measurements the free carriers were identified as electrons, and so it would appear that the free holes were quickly trapped by the boron centres. This could account for the long decay time, in the dark, of the E.S.R. signal.

Under illumination the steady-state concentration of electrons is given by

$$n_e = G\tau \tag{6.1}$$

where G is the rate of production of electron-hole pairs and τ is the electron-hole recombination time. Bemski and Szymanski[1] estimated 10^{-9} sec $< \tau < 10^{-8}$ sec and, from a knowledge of the donor-impurity concentration, estimated that the cross-section for the capture of electrons at neutral acceptors is $\sim 10^{-14}$ cm^2 at $1\cdot2°$K.

In a compensated sample of n-type silicon ($N_d > N_a$) at liquid helium temperatures, and under equilibrium conditions

$$N_d^0 = N_d - N_a \qquad (6.2a)$$

$$N_d^+ = N_a^- \qquad (6.2b)$$

$$N_a^- = N_a \qquad (6.2c)$$

where N_d^0 is the concentration of neutral donor impurities, and N_d^+ and N_a^- are the concentrations of ionized donor-impurity centres and negative acceptor ions respectively. If such a sample is illuminated by intrinsic radiation, then the resultant free electrons and holes are quickly captured by the ionized donor impurities and the negative acceptor ions respectively. The intensity of the E.S.R. signal is proportional to N_d^0, and if the creation of electron-hole pairs is greater than the transfer rate for electrons from donor to acceptor impurities, then $N_d^0 \simeq N_d$. Initially the E.S.R. signal is proportional to N_d^0 as given by the equation (6.2a), so the signal should increase in intensity by the factor $(1 - N_a/N_d)^{-1}$. In this way the compensation ratio N_a/N_d can be measured directly.

Honig and Levitt[2] measured the ratio of the capture cross-section for free electrons at positively ionized donor centres and neutral acceptor centres in a silicon sample with $N_d = 5 \times 10^{15}$ cm^{-3} (phosphorus) and $N_a = 2 \cdot 5 \times 10^{15}$ cm^{-3} (boron). Extrinsic radiation was used to delocalize the donor electrons[3] and the differential equations governing the rates of change of the concentrations of neutral donors and free electrons are

$$\frac{dN_d^0}{dt} = -S_d N_d^0 + \sigma_d^+ (N_d - N_d^0) n_e \qquad (6.3a)$$

$$\frac{dn_e}{dt} = S_d N_d^0 - \sigma_d^+ (N_d - N_d^0) n_e - \sigma_a^0 N_a^0 n_e \qquad (6.3b)$$

where S_d is the rate of ionization of neutral donor impurities, $(N_d - N_d^0)$ equals the concentration of positively ionized donor impurities, and σ_d^+ and σ_a^0 are the capture cross-sections for electrons of the positively ionized donor impurities and the neutral acceptor impurities respectively. By fitting the solutions of equations (6.3) to the observed concentration of neutral donor impurities, Honig and Levitt found $\sigma_a{}^0/\sigma_a{}^+ = 3\cdot2\times10^{-2}$ to an accuracy of 50 per cent.

In a sample of silicon with 5×10^{16} phosphorus atoms cm^{-3} and $2\cdot5\times10^{16}$ boron atoms cm^{-3} illumination with intrinsic radiation at $4\cdot2°K$ decreases the dark conductivity by a factor of five. As this is attributed to the filling of positively ionized donor centres, it means that there is a decrease in the possibility of electron 'hopping' processes which give rise to impurity conduction in compensated samples of this impurity concentration.[4]

§6.2

SURFACE STATES

As was mentioned in §2.4, an additional resonance line ($g \simeq 2\cdot006$, line width 6 to 8 gauss) is observed in n-type silicon samples powdered in air. This line is attributed to paramagnetic centres associated with the damaged surfaces of the particles.[5] A similar line has also been observed in powdered samples of germanium and in single-crystal specimens of both n-type and p-type silicon whose surfaces had been sand blasted.[6,7,8]

The line disappears after etching with suitable solutions* which remove about one micron of the surface. Feher[8] subjected samples to cycles of etching and sand blasting and found that the resonance line was reproducible. It was, in fact, noted that more than one line could be observed,[9] depending on the conditions of ambient temperature and gas pressure, and on the nature of the ambient atmosphere, both during and subsequent to the powdering process.

If high purity n- or p-type silicon is carefully etched, transferred immediately to an ultra-high vacuum system ($\sim10^{-9}$ torr), and then crushed, no E.S.R. signal is observed[9] (to within the spectrometer sensitivity: $\sim10^{12}\Delta H$ spins/gauss).

For silicon crushed in air, sealed in quartz tubes at 10^{-5} torr pressure, and subsequently heated to between $400°C$ and $700°C$, a line $0\cdot8$ gauss wide with a g-value $2\cdot0024$ was observed by Kusumoto and Shoji.[10]

Müller *et al.*[9] carried out a series of experiments, under carefully controlled conditions of ambient gas pressure and temperature, to

---

* For example, 30 parts HF, 50 parts HNO_3, 30 parts CH_3COOH, and 1 part Br. The rate of reaction is more controllable if the solution is kept at $0°C$.

determine the characteristics of the surface state resonances. Their results may be summarized as follows. A narrow line, corresponding to that observed by Kusumoto and Shoji, is observed for low oxygen content near the silicon surface. For increasing oxygen content, the line width and g-value increase until, for silicon crushed in air and not subjected to vacuum treatment, the values are 6 to 8 gauss and $2 \cdot 0055$ respectively. It is worthy of note that, for bulk silicon monoxide, the E.S.R. line width is 7 gauss and the g-value[9] is $2 \cdot 0049$. Feher[8] ascribed the lines to aggregates of oxygen, and Müller *et al.* proposed that these aggregates diffused into the silicon during the heat treatment following the crushing process. From the line width measurements it was concluded that the line broadening mechanism is due to dipolar interaction between paramagnetic oxygen physically adsorbed at the surface and the paramagnetic centres produced near the surface. Hence, assuming that the relaxation rates $1/T_1$ and $1/T_2$ are proportional to the number of adsorbed oxygen molecules per cm^2, the change in line width is given by

$$\Delta H - \Delta H_0 = KN \qquad (6.4)$$

where K is a constant and N is the number of adsorbed oxygen molecules per cm^2.

According to Müller *et al.*, there is a logarithmic dependence of N on the oxygen partial pressure; the observed line widths are consistent with this. For an atmosphere of 100 per cent oxygen, the rate of change of line width with pressure is three times as great as for atmospheres containing up to only 20 per cent oxygen.

§6.3

NUCLEAR POLARIZATION SCHEMES

Interest in nuclear polarization schemes has arisen mainly, perhaps, from the usefulness to nuclear physicists of targets containing oriented nuclei. Although high energy experiments of fundamental interest required polarized targets of protons or deuterons, samples of semiconductors, such as silicon and indium antimonide, containing oriented heavy nuclei are also of some interest. Apart from scattering experiments, information may also be obtained concerning nuclear decay modes, parity non-conservation, the angular distribution of α-, β-, and γ-rays, and on nuclear spins and magnetic moments.

The various polarization schemes are of interest also from the point of view of 'spin-pumping', i.e. the re-arrangement of the populations of energy-level systems by means of resonant radiation.

Nuclear polarizations are of interest for cooling experiments in the microdegree region, since they correspond to low spin temperatures.

Silicon has proved to be a very fruitful field for experiments of this kind, the principal reason being the length of the relaxation times of the donor electrons and of the donor and Si^{29} nuclei.

For an assembly of N nuclei of spin I in a magnetic field H the polarization can be taken to be

$$P = \frac{\langle I_z \rangle}{I} \tag{6.5}$$

Here $\langle I_z \rangle$ is the average value of I in the direction of the applied magnetic field and, of course, I is the maximum value which the component of I in the direction of H can take. In the general case

$$P = \frac{\sum_m m N_m}{I \sum_m N_m} \tag{6.6}$$

where m is the magnetic quantum number labelling the $(2I+1)$ energy levels and N_m is the number of nuclei in the mth state.

For $I = \frac{1}{2}$, such as for phosphorus in silicon, there are two nuclear states, and if N_+, N_- are the numbers of nuclei with spin 'up' and spin 'down' respectively, then, at thermal equilibrium,

$$P = \frac{N_+ - N_-}{N_+ + N_-} = \frac{1 - \exp(-g_N \beta_N H/kT)}{1 + \exp(-g_N \beta_N H/kT)}$$

$$= \tanh g_N \beta_N H/2kT \simeq g_N \beta_N H/2kT \equiv \Delta_N \tag{6.7}$$

i.e. the polarization is determined by the nuclear Boltzmann factor. Typically this yields values for the polarization of 10^{-5} at liquid helium temperatures for magnetic fields of a few thousand gauss.

Overhauser[11] considered the hyperfine coupling between conduction electrons and nuclei in metals, and suggested that through saturation of the E.S.R. signal at microwave frequencies an appreciable polarization of the nuclei could be obtained. Such an enhanced polarization was subsequently observed.[12] In fact, it was soon realized that this principle could be extended to a large number of coupled electron-nuclear systems,[13] the necessary condition being that the nuclei relax via the electrons whose spins are being saturated.

Consider a system of nuclear spins in fluctuating contact due to thermal vibrations, with a system of electron spins. For simplicity we will consider $I = \frac{1}{2}$. If $N_{\pm}$, $n_{\pm}$ are the numbers of nuclear spins and electron spins respectively pointing parallel and antiparallel to the magnetic field, then, for mutual electron-nuclear spin flips,

$$\frac{dN_-}{dt} = -\frac{N_- n_+}{N}W(+ - \;\rightarrow\; - +) + \frac{N_+ n_-}{N}W(- + \;\rightarrow\; + -)$$

$$(6.8)$$

where N is the total number of nuclei and W represents transition probabilities for the transitions induced by lattice vibrations.*

$$\frac{W(- + \;\rightarrow\; + -)}{W(+ - \;\rightarrow\; - +)} = \exp[-(g\beta - g_N\beta_N)H/kT_L] \qquad (6.9)$$

since these transitions establish the thermal equilibrium level populations at the lattice temperature T_L.

In the steady state $dN_-/dt = 0$ and from equations (6.8) and (6.9)

$$\frac{N_+}{N_-} = \frac{n_+}{n_-} \exp[(g\beta - g_N\beta_N)H/kT_L] \qquad (6.10)$$

Now the electron spin temperature T_s and nuclear spin temperature T_N are defined through

$$\frac{n_+}{n_-} = \exp(-g\beta H/kT_s) \qquad (6.11)$$

---

* Lattice here strictly means environment, since these arguments are not restricted to solids.

9

and

$$\frac{N_+}{N_-} = \exp(-g_N\beta_N H/kT_N) \tag{6.12}$$

Thus, on substituting for n_+/n_- and N_+/N_- in equation (6.10), we obtain

$$\frac{1}{T_N} = \frac{g\beta}{g_N\beta_N}\left(\frac{1}{T_s} - \frac{1}{T_L}\right) + \frac{1}{T_L} \tag{6.13}$$

If $T_s = T_L$, then $1/T_N = 1/T_L$ and the nuclear polarization is just equal to the thermal equilibrium value.

If, however, the E.S.R. transition is saturated then $T_s \to \infty$ and

$$1/T_N \simeq 1/T_L(1 - g\beta/g_N\beta_N)$$

As $g\beta/g_N\beta_N \sim 10^3$, the nuclear spin temperature is negative, corresponding to a large, negative, nuclear polarization. We see that now the magnitude of the nuclear polarization is related to the electronic Boltzmann factor [compare with equation (6.7)]. The nuclear polarization can be determined from the amplitude of the nuclear resonance signal, which is proportional to P.

It is also noteworthy that an enhanced nuclear polarization can be obtained in the following way. Suppose the kinetic energy of the electrons can be made larger than the thermal equilibrium value appropriate to the lattice temperature. Call this higher temperature T_R. Then in equation (6.9) T_L is replaced by T_R and in equation (6.11) T_s is replaced by T_L, since it is assumed that the electron spins retain their thermal equilibrium distribution. So now in equation (6.13) we have, since $T_R \to \infty$, $1/T_N = g\beta/g_N\beta_N \cdot 1/T_L$ and again an enhanced nuclear polarization is obtained (of different sign, note). This enhanced polarization can be obtained without the aid of microwave fields. Electrons whose kinetic energy is greater than the thermal equilibrium value are known as 'hot' electrons (see p. 128).

In practice there are other relaxation processes apart from the electron-nuclear interaction which produce 'leakage' effects, and the actual enhanced nuclear polarizations obtained are somewhat less than the values predicted by this simple treatment of the problem.[14]

Dynamic nuclear polarization using radio frequency fields

As we are concerned with semiconductors, we shall consider nuclear polarization effects in the simple situation of a donor electron coupled to a phosphorus nuclei ($I = \frac{1}{2}$) in silicon, at liquid helium temperatures.

The spin Hamiltonian is

$$\mathscr{H} = g\beta \mathbf{S} . \mathbf{H} + a\mathbf{S} . \mathbf{I} - g_N \beta_N \mathbf{I} . \mathbf{H} \qquad (6.14)$$

and the energy levels are given by

$$E(m_s, m_I) = g\beta H m_s + a m_s m_I \qquad (6.15)$$

Here the nuclear Zeeman term has been neglected in comparison with the hyperfine interaction term. The energy-level diagram and the relative populations of the levels at thermal equilibrium, together with relaxation processes, are shown in Fig. 6.2(a) where $\Delta \equiv g\beta H/2kT$ and $\delta = a/4kT$. The nuclear polarization is, according to equation (6.6), given by

$$P = \frac{\frac{1}{2}\{\exp[-2(\Delta+\delta)]+1\} - \frac{1}{2}[\exp(-2\Delta)+\exp(-2\delta)]}{\frac{1}{2}\{1+\exp[-2(\Delta+\delta)]+\exp(-2\Delta)+\exp(-2\delta)\}}$$
$$\simeq \delta\Delta \qquad (6.16)$$

which is of the order of 10^{-5}.

If the 1 to 2 electronic transition is saturated and thermal equilibrium is established between the populations of levels 2, 3 and 4, then a nuclear polarization can be obtained.[15] Taking as unity the equal populations of levels 1 and 2 [see Fig. 6.2(b)], it follows that $P \simeq \Delta/2$. This is the Overhauser effect.

The 2 to 4 transition involves a mutual electron-nuclear spin flip $[\Delta(m_s + m_I) = 0]$ and is forbidden in the first order. However, if there is sufficient radio frequency power available to induce these transitions at a greater rate than the relaxation rate, then the transition can be saturated [see Fig. 6.2(c)]. Assuming that the electron spin-lattice interaction is the dominant relaxation process, then the level populations are as shown in Fig. 6.2(c) and $P \simeq -\Delta$. This polarization scheme has been employed in experiments to measure the spins and magnetic moments of the radio-active nuclei As^{76} and Sb^{122} (see §6.5).

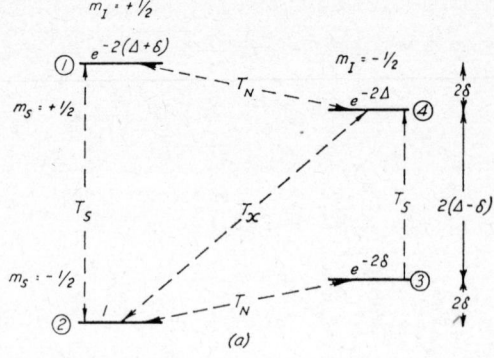

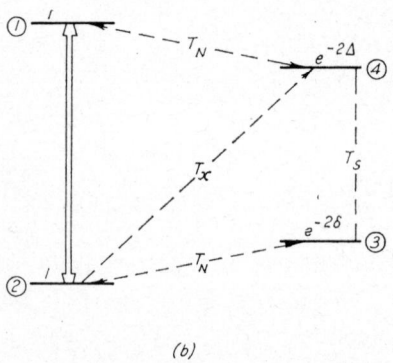

FIG. 6.2. (a) The energy levels for an electron coupled to a nucleus having a spin $I = \frac{1}{2}$. The relative populations of the levels and the various relaxation processes are also indicated.
(b) The scheme for obtaining a nuclear polarization $P \simeq \Delta/2$ by saturating one of the $\Delta m_s = \pm 1$ electronic transitions.

The foregoing elementary arguments illustrate the general features of the polarization schemes, but for more detailed information on, for instance, partial saturation and transient behaviour, the rate equations for the system must be solved.[14]

Feher[16] showed that nuclear polarizations could be obtained in systems showing resolved hyperfine lines, subject to two conditions. Firstly, it must be possible to traverse the resonance transitions

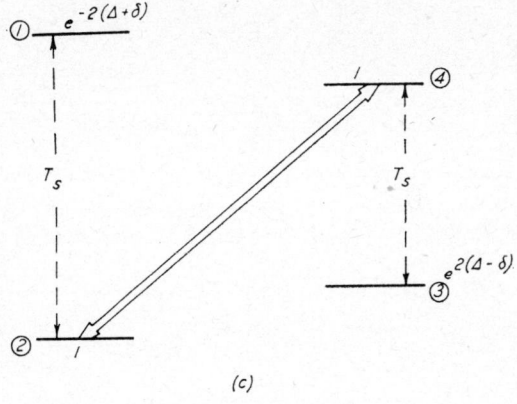

(c)

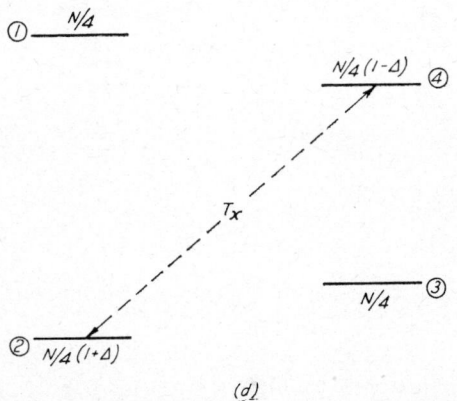

(d)

FIG. 6.2. (c) The scheme for obtaining a nuclear polarization $P \simeq -\Delta$ by saturating the first order forbidden electronic transition $\Delta(m_s + m_I) = 0$ between levels 2 and 4.
(d) $T_x \ll T_s$: If the magnetic field is increased from zero to a steady value, then a polarization $P \simeq \Delta/2$ will be established which will persist for a time of the order of T_s. This scheme does not involve the use of a microwave field.

(both electronic and nuclear) under 'abiabatic fast passage' conditions.[17,18] Secondly, the difference between the nuclear transition frequencies, predicted by the Breit–Rabi formula,[19,20] (see Fig. 6.3), should be greater than the nuclear resonance line widths. This allows one nuclear resonance transition to be excited

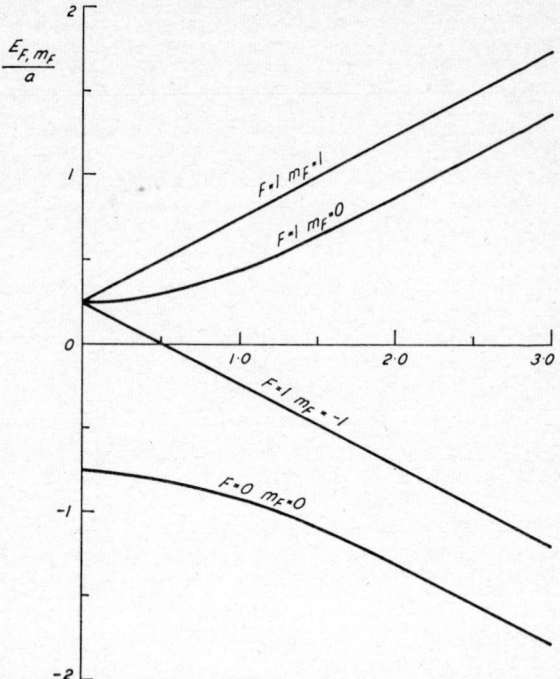

FIG. 6.3. The energy levels as a function of applied magnetic field for a system consisting of an electron coupled to a nucleus of spin $I = \frac{1}{2}$, as predicted by the Breit–Rabi formula.[19,20] $\mathbf{F} = \mathbf{J} + \mathbf{I}$. a is the hyperfine interaction constant and $x = (g_J + g_I)\beta H/a$.

independently of the others. In the process of abiabatic fast passage through a resonance line, the line is swept through in a time less than the relaxation time and the important result is that the populations of the two levels are inverted.

Consider phosphorus-doped silicon (see Fig. 6.4). If the populations of levels 1 and 2 are inverted by adiabatic fast passage through the electronic transition, and subsequently the populations of levels 1 and 4 are inverted by adiabatic fast passage through the nuclear transition, then a nuclear polarization of approximate magnitude Δ should be established. Feher and Gere[21] used the E.S.R. signal as a probe to investigate the level populations and verified that nuclear polarizations could be obtained by this method.

The magnetic field determining Δ can be considerably higher than that at which the electronic and nuclear transitions are induced, providing it is reduced to the value at resonance in a time much less than the relaxation times.

Feher and Gere used a magnetic field in the region of 3100 gauss and the nuclear transition frequencies were between 52 and 54 Mc/s, and 64 and 66 Mc/s respectively.

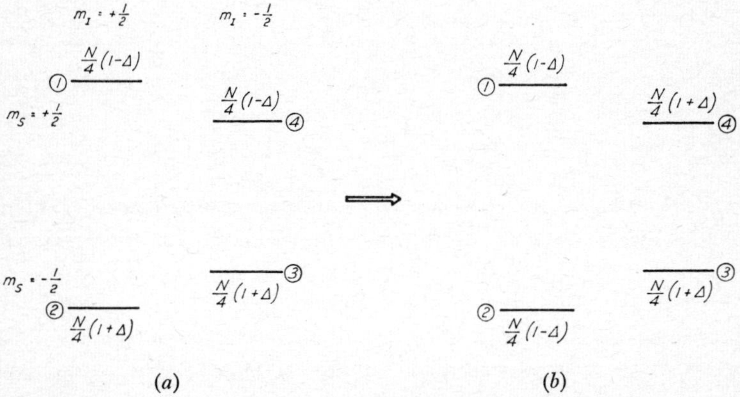

FIG. 6.4. A scheme for obtaining a nuclear polarization of magnitude Δ for an electron coupled to a phosphorus nucleus in silicon.
(a) The populations of levels 1 and 2 are inverted by an adiabatic fast passage through the resonance magnetic field.
(b) Subsequently the populations of levels 1 and 4 are inverted by adiabatic fast passage through the relevant nuclear transition.

Abragam *et al.*[22] observed dynamic polarization of the Si^{29} nuclei in *n*-type silicon (5×10^{16} phosphorus atoms cm^{-3}) at $77°$K. At this temperature the donor-impurity centres are ionized and the electrons are in the conduction band, i.e. they are delocalized. Thus, only the isotropic Fermi contact term need be considered for the hyperfine interaction. Among the advantages of using such samples of silicon, compared with metals, is that, firstly, the skin depth for the microwave radiation is much greater (~ 100 microns as compared with ~ 1 micron for copper) and, secondly, because of the low concentration of conduction electrons, the nuclear relaxation times are longer ($\sim$ minutes for samples with a free carrier concentration $\sim 10^{17}$ cm^{-3}).[23] Abragam *et al.* saturated the $\Delta(m_s + m_I) = 0$ transitions, using an X-band magnetron (8 watts), and obtained enhancements of the nuclear resonance signal, which is proportional to the nuclear polarization, of the order of 100.

Other nuclear polarization schemes

In this section we will mention two polarization schemes which do not require a microwave field to saturate an E.S.R. line. This obviously makes for a much simpler polarization scheme from the point of view of the nuclear physicist.

Consider first phosphorus-doped silicon [see Fig. 6.2(a)]. Under certain conditions T_x may be the dominant relaxation process. The magnetic field is increased from zero to a steady value and then kept constant for a time greater than T_x but less than T_s. Thermal equilibrium will be established between levels 4 and 2, the populations being as shown in Fig. 6.2(b). Hence, a polarization of $\Delta/2$ is established which will persist for a time of the order of T_s.[14,15] The reduction of T_x with applied stress is obviously an important factor in this effect.[16]

We have indicated earlier how a nuclear polarization can be obtained in a semiconductor sample containing 'hot' electrons. Clark and Feher[24] have investigated this phenomenon in silicon and indium antimonide. The existence of hot electrons can be detected by departures from Ohm's law when an electric field is applied.

Feher[25] carried out experiments on silicon (phosphorus-doped: $N_d = 2 \times 10^{16}$ cm^{-3}, $N_a = 8 \times 10^{14}$ cm^{-3}) at 1·3°K and established that for the electrons bound to the phosphorus nuclei, T_s increased to approximately 2·6°K as T_R was increased to the order of 100°K (electric field = 6 volt/cm). It was assumed that the bound electrons relaxed through spin exchange with the conduction electrons and that therefore the spin temperature of the two systems of electrons attained the same value (see p. 43).

Optical excitation was used to introduce conduction electrons ($10^8 - 10^{10}$ cm^{-3}) and the electric field was applied through suitable n^+ electrodes.[26]

Because of the small number of conduction electrons, the actual nuclear polarization produced was small.

The situation should be more favourable in semiconductors having a higher electron mobility, since higher current densities can be used without heating appreciably the sample. Clark and Feher[24] have observed enhanced nuclear polarizations, using the hot electron technique, in indium antimonide where the electron mobility is very high ($\sim 5 \times 10^4$ cm^2/volt . sec).

In experiments at $4 \cdot 2°$K on a sample having a conduction electron concentration of 4×10^{15} cm^{-3} enhancement factors (T_L/T_N) of $4 \cdot 2$, $9 \cdot 0$, and $11 \cdot 8$ were observed, through their nuclear resonances, for In^{115}, Sb^{121}, and Sb^{123} respectively. The applied electric field was $0 \cdot 9$ volt/cm.

It was calculated that the conduction electron-nuclear relaxation time should be of the order of 100 hours for In^{115} and Sb^{121}, whereas the observed total nuclear relaxation times were $3 \cdot 5$ hours and 5 hours respectively. This appears to indicate that there are 'leakage' relaxation processes probably due to interactions between the nuclei and paramagnetic impurities. If the concentration of the latter could be reduced, then the nuclear polarizations could be correspondingly increased.

§6.4

INVESTIGATION OF THE HYPERFINE STRUCTURE ANOMALY

As was mentioned in Chapter 2, hyperfine interaction constants can be measured with great accuracy by the E.N.D.O.R. technique. Eisinger and Feher[27] have made use of this feature of the technique to measure the hyperfine structure anomaly for the stable isotopes of antimony (Sb^{121} and Sb^{123}).

The Fermi–Segrè expression[28] for the 'contact' hyperfine interaction was calculated on the assumption that the nucleus can be represented by a point dipole. In a more precise calculation account must be taken of the distribution of the magnetic moment inside the nucleus and of the modification of the electron wave function inside the nucleus.

The modified expression for the hyperfine interaction constant can be written in the form,[27]

$$a = \frac{8\pi}{3} g g_N \beta \beta_N |\psi(0)|^2 (1 + C_1)(1 + C_2) \qquad (6.17)$$

Here the correction term $(1 + C_1)$ is related to the distribution of magnetic moment in the nucleus,[29] and the term $(1 + C_2)$ is related to the modification of the electron wave function inside the nucleus.[30]

Thus, for the two isotopes of antimony, it follows that

$$\frac{a_{121}}{a_{123}} = \frac{g_{121}}{g_{123}}(1 + \Lambda_1 + \Lambda_2) \tag{6.18}$$

where $\Lambda_1 = C_1^{121} - C_1^{123}$ and $\Lambda_2 = C_2^{121} - C_2^{123}$.

The measured hyperfine structure anomaly Λ is defined through

$$\Lambda = \left(\frac{a_{121}}{a_{123}}\right)\left(\frac{g_{123}}{g_{121}}\right) - 1 \tag{6.19}$$

In fact, it is found that Λ_2 is much smaller than Λ_1 (by a factor $\sim 10^2$).

Eisinger and Feher found a value of -0.352 ± 0.005 per cent for Λ_1, and compared this result with calculated values based on four nuclear models.

It was not expected that the fact that the theories referred to free atoms, whilst the experiments were performed on atoms in the solid, would lead to difficulties when comparing results. There are two main reasons for this. Firstly, it is the ratio of the hyperfine interactions which is of interest. Secondly, the behaviour of an electron inside the nucleus, where the 'contact' hyperfine interaction arises, will be essentially the same whether the nucleus is in a free atom or in an atom in a solid.

The nuclear models used in the comparison were the extreme single particle model, the collective model, the single particle-uniform interpolation model, and the configuration mixing model.[31] On the basis of this comparison only the single particle-uniform interpolation model gives a result (-0.72 per cent) differing widely from the experimental value (see Table III of Eisinger and Feher[27]).

§6.5

THE MEASUREMENT OF NUCLEAR MAGNETIC MOMENTS

The E.N.D.O.R. technique can be used to measure nuclear magnetic moments in systems for which the frequencies of the nuclear transitions ($\Delta m_s = 0$, $\Delta m_I = \pm 1$) for states of different m_s are different, and for which the frequency difference is greater than the nuclear resonance line widths. This is perhaps best illustrated by reference to a system for which $S = \frac{1}{2}$ and $I = \frac{1}{2}$. The difference between the nuclear transition frequencies can be calculated from the Breit–Rabi formula.[19] In a magnetic field H the energy levels are given by

$$E_{F,m_F} = -\frac{a}{4} + g_I\beta H m_F \pm \frac{a}{2}(1 + 2m_F x + x^2)^{1/2} \qquad (6.20)$$

where the $+$ and $-$ signs refer to the situations with $F = 1$ and 0 respectively; m_F can take the values $F, F-1, \ldots -F$ (see Fig. 6.3) and

$$x \equiv (g_J + g_I)\frac{\beta H}{a} \qquad (6.21)$$

Here $g_I = g_N \cdot m_e/M_N$ is the modified nuclear g-factor.

It follows that

$$h\nu' - h\nu = 2g_I\beta H + a(1 + x^2)^{1/2} - ax \qquad (6.22)$$

The frequencies ν', ν can be measured very accurately by the E.N.D.O.R. technique and a value for g_I calculated. Hence, an absolute value of the nuclear magnetic moment can be obtained. The important feature of this method is that the value of the electron wave function at the nucleus is not required.

Feher *et al.*[32] measured the nuclear spin and nuclear magnetic moment of 14-day P^{32} in silicon. The sample contained 8×10^{16} P^{31} atoms cm^{-3} and $1 \cdot 6 \times 10^{15}$ P^{32} atoms cm^{-3}. In fact, the observed P^{32} lines lay under and between the 'satellite' lines due to pairs and clusters of three P^{31} atoms (see pp. 31 to 33). Nevertheless, from the spacing of the two extreme P^{32} lines (equal to $2aI$), the value of I was found to be unity.

The nuclear g-factor for P^{32} was calculated from the expression

$$\frac{a(P^{32})}{a(P^{31})} = \frac{g(P^{32})}{g(P^{31})}(1 + \Lambda) \qquad (6.23)$$

where the hyperfine structure anomaly Λ was calculated to be $+0 \cdot 17$ per cent, yielding

$$g(P^{32}) = -0 \cdot 2523 \pm 0 \cdot 0003 \qquad (6.24)$$

The sign of the nuclear magnetic moment was determined by saturating one of the electronic transitions and observing the relative amplitudes of the E.N.D.O.R. lines.[32]

Culvahouse, Pipkin, and others[33,34,35] have measured the nuclear spins and magnetic moments of the radioactive isotopes As^{76} and Sb^{122}. The nuclei were first polarized by saturating a forbidden electronic transition in which the electron and nuclear spins are simultaneously flipped. This method relies on there being sufficient microwave power available to saturate the forbidden transition and this is indeed the case for many systems in the liquid helium temperature range.[14] The nuclear polarization was detected by observing the anisotropy of the emitted γ-rays, as the large magnetic field was varied, by means of a thallium-activated, sodium iodide scintillation counter. The sensitivity inherent in this technique derives from the fact that the changes of direction of γ-ray photons are detected by a *quantum* detector.

§6.6

A TWO-LEVEL MASER

If the thermal equilibrium magnetization of a spin system, contained in a microwave cavity, is inverted, then the condition for spontaneous radiation of the stored energy into the cavity is:[36]

$$N \geqslant kTV_c\Delta H \langle H_c^2 \rangle / 4\pi Q\beta^2 H_o \langle H_s^2 \rangle \qquad (6.25)$$

Here N is the total number of spins, V_c and Q are the volume and loaded Q-factor respectively of the microwave cavity, ΔH is the width of the E.S.R. line, H_o is the steady magnetic field at resonance, and $\langle H_c^2 \rangle$ and $\langle H_s^2 \rangle$ are the squares of the microwave magnetic field averaged over the volume of the cavity and the volume of the sample respectively.

The population inversion can be obtained in phosphorus-doped silicon by an adiabatic fast passage through one of the phosphorus hyperfine lines. However, Combrisson *et al.*[36] were unable to obtain maser oscillations in ordinary phosphorus-doped silicon where $\Delta H = 2\cdot7$ gauss.

Since this line width is due to hyperfine interactions with the 5 per cent naturally abundant Si^{29} nuclei (see §2.1), Feher *et al.*[37] employed an isotopically enriched silicon sample (99·88 per cent

Si[28]) in which ΔH was reduced by an order of magnitude to 0·22 gauss. They obtained maser oscillations in a cavity which had a Q-factor of about 20 000.

Of course, being a two-level maser, the output of radiation is not continuous. The level populations are inverted and made to radiate coherently into the cavity by successive sweeps of the magnetic field backwards and forwards through the resonance value.

References

1. Bemski, G., and Szymanski, B., *J. Phys. Chem. Solids*, 1960, **17**, 173.
2. Honig, A., and Levitt, R., *Phys. Rev. Letters*, 1960, **5**, 93.
3. Spitzer, W., and Fan, H. Y., *Phys. Rev.*, 1957, **108**, 268.
4. Mott, N. F., and Twose, W. D., *Adv. in Physics*, 1961, **10**, 107.
5. Lancaster, G., and Schneider, E. E., *Proc. Int. Conf. on Semiconductor Physics*, p. 589 (Czech. Acad. of Sci., 1961).
6. Walters, G. K., *J. Phys. Chem. Solids*, 1960, **14**, 43.
7. Fletcher, R. C., Yager, W. A., Pearson, G. L., Holden, A. N., and Merritt, F. R., *Phys. Rev.*, 1954, **94**, 1392.
8. Feher, G., *Phys. Rev.*, 1959, **114**, 1219.
9. Müller, K. A., Chan, P., Kleiner, R., Ovenall, D. W., and Sparnaay, M. J., *J. Appl. Phys.*, 1964, **35**, 2254.
10. Kusomoto, H., and Shoji, M., *J. Phys. Soc., Japan*, 1962, **17**, 1678.
11. Overhauser, A., *Phys. Rev.*, 1953, **92**, 411.
12. Carver, T. R., and Slichter, C. P., *Phys. Rev.*, 1956, **102**, 975.
13. Abragam, A., *Phys. Rev.*, 1955, **98**, 1729.
14. See, for instance, Jeffries, C. D., *Dynamic Nuclear Orientation*, (Interscience Tracts, 1963).
15. Pines, D., Bardeen, J., and Slichter, C. P., *Phys. Rev.*, 1957, **106**, 489.
16. Feher, G., *Phys. Rev.*, 1956, **103**, 500.
17. Bloch, F., *Phys. Rev.*, 1946, **70**, 460.
18. Abragam, A., *The Principles of Nuclear Magnetism*, Chapter 3 (Oxford, 1961).
19. Breit, G., and Rabi, I. I., *Phys. Rev.*, 1940, **38**, 2082.
20. Kisch, P., Millman, S., and Rabi, I. I., *Phys. Rev.*, 1940, **57**, 765.
21. Feher, G., and Gere, E. A., *Phys. Rev.*, 1956, **103**, 501.
22. Abragam, A., Combrisson, J., and Solomon, I., *C. R. Acad. Sci.*, 1958, **246**, 1035.
23. Shulman, R. G., and Wyluda, B. L., *Phys. Rev.*, 1956, **103**, 1127.
24. Clark, W. G., and Feher, G., *Phys. Rev. Letters,* 1963, **10**, 134.
25. Feher, G., *Phys. Rev. Letters*, 1959, **3**, 135.
26. Smith, R. A., *Semiconductors*, Chapter 8 (Cambridge, 1961).
27. Eisinger, J., and Feher, G., *Phys. Rev.*, 1958, **109**, 1172.
28. Fermi, E., and Segrè, E. G., *Z. Phys.*, 1933, **82**, 729.
29. Bohr, A., and Weisskopf, V. F., *Phys. Rev.*, 1950, **77**, 94.
30. Rosenthal, J. E., and Breit, G., *Phys. Rev.*, 1932, **41**, 459.
31. Blin-Stoyle, R. J., *Rev. Mod. Phys.*, 1956, **28**, 92.
32. Feher, G., Fuller, C. S., and Gere, E. A., *Phys. Rev.*, 1957, **107**, 1462.
33. Pipkin, F. M., and Culvahouse, J. W., *Phys. Rev.*, 1957, **106**, 1102.
34. Pipkin, F. M., *Phys. Rev.*, 1958, **112**, 935.

35. Bradley, G. E., Pipkin, F. M., and Simpson, R. E., *Phys. Rev.*, 1961, **123**, 1824.
36. Combrisson, J., Honig, A., and Townes, C. H., *C. R. Acad. Sci.*, 1956, **242**, 2451.
37. Feher, G., Gordon, J. P., Buehler, E., Gere, E. A., and Thurmond, C. D., *Phys. Rev.*, 1958, **109**, 221.

Appendix

WANNIER FUNCTIONS AND SHALLOW
DONOR-IMPURITY STATES

In a perfect crystal the motion of electrons can be described by Bloch functions. These are non-localized functions and the position of a particular electron is not specified. If we are interested in a perturbation problem associated with a particular locality in a crystal, such as an isolated impurity centre, then the wave function can be written as a combination of Bloch functions.

$$\chi = \sum_n \sum_k C_n(\mathbf{k})\psi_{n,\mathbf{k}}(\mathbf{r}) \qquad (1)$$

Here n is the band index and $\psi_{n,r,\mathbf{k}}(\mathbf{r})$ is a Bloch function in the nth band. This equation is not easy to deal with if a number of coefficients C_n are required to give a good description of the electron wave function in the perturbed situation.

Wannier defined localized functions, $a_n(\mathbf{r}-\mathbf{l})$, which are derived from the true Bloch functions, in the following way:

$$\psi_{n,\mathbf{k}}(\mathbf{r}) \equiv \frac{1}{\sqrt{N}}\sum_l \exp[i\mathbf{k}.\mathbf{l}.a_n(\mathbf{r}-\mathbf{l})] \qquad (2)$$

where $\mathbf{l}$ is the vector to a lattice site and N is the number of atoms in the crystal. If we multiply equation (1) by $\exp(-i\mathbf{k} . \mathbf{l}')$ and sum over the N values of $\mathbf{k}$, then we have:

$$\sum_k \exp(-i\mathbf{k}.\mathbf{l}')\psi_{n,\mathbf{k}}(\mathbf{r}) = \frac{1}{\sqrt{N}}\sum_l \sum_k \exp[i\mathbf{k}.(\mathbf{l}-\mathbf{l}')a_n(\mathbf{r}-\mathbf{l})]$$

$$= \sqrt{N}\sum_l a_n(\mathbf{r}-\mathbf{l})\delta_{\mathbf{l},\mathbf{l}'}$$

$$= \sqrt{N}a_n(\mathbf{r}-\mathbf{l}') \qquad (3)$$

Thus we can write

$$a_n(\mathbf{r}-\mathbf{l}) = \frac{1}{\sqrt{N}}\sum_{\mathbf{k}} \exp(-i\mathbf{k}.\mathbf{l})\psi_{n,\mathbf{k}}(\mathbf{r}) \tag{4}$$

The localized nature of Wannier functions is illustrated by using the example of a simple cubic lattice (side of unit cell $= d_0$) and by making the approximation that $u_\mathbf{k}(\mathbf{r})$ in the Bloch function $\psi_{n,\mathbf{k}}(\mathbf{r}) = \exp(i\mathbf{k}.\mathbf{r})u_\mathbf{k}(\mathbf{r})$ is independent of $\mathbf{k}$. For a large crystal $\Sigma_\mathbf{k}$ may be replaced by an integral, the density of k-values being $V/8\pi^3 = N/8 \cdot (d_0/\pi)^3$. Then

$$a_n(\mathbf{r}-\mathbf{l}) = \frac{\sqrt{N}}{8}\left(\frac{d_0}{\pi}\right)^3 u_n(\mathbf{r}) \iiint \exp[-ik_x(x-x_l)]$$

$$\exp[-ik_y(y-y_l)] \exp[-ik_z(z-z_l)]dk_x\, dk_y\, dk_z \tag{5}$$

where the limits of integration are $k_x, k_y, k_z = -\pi/d_0$ to π/d_0, $\mathbf{r} = \mathbf{i}x+\mathbf{j}y+\mathbf{k}z$ and $\mathbf{l} = \mathbf{i}x_l+\mathbf{j}y_l+\mathbf{k}z_l$. From (5) we have

$$a_n(\mathbf{r}-\mathbf{l}) = \sqrt{N}u_n(\mathbf{r})$$

$$\times\frac{[\sin\pi(x-x_l)/d_0]\,[\sin\pi(y-y_l)/d_0]\,[\sin\pi(z-z_l)/d_0]}{(x-x_l)(y-y_l)(z-z_l)(\pi/d_0)^3} \tag{6}$$

and we see that $|a_n(\mathbf{r}-\mathbf{l})|^2$ looks like

$$|u_n(\mathbf{r})|^2 \frac{\sin^2\pi(x-x_l)/d_0}{[\pi(x-x_l)/d_0]^2}$$

(see Fig. 1) in the x-direction and similarly in the y- and z-directions. Now

$$\int a_n^*(\mathbf{r}-\mathbf{l})a_n(\mathbf{r}-\mathbf{l}')d\mathbf{r}$$

$$= \frac{1}{N}\int \sum_\mathbf{k}\exp(i\mathbf{k}.\mathbf{l})\psi_{n,\mathbf{k}}^*(\mathbf{r})\sum_{\mathbf{k}'}\exp(-i\mathbf{k}'.\mathbf{l}')\psi_{n,\mathbf{k}'}(\mathbf{r})\,d\mathbf{r}$$

$$= \frac{1}{N}\sum_\mathbf{k}\sum_{\mathbf{k}'}\exp(i\mathbf{k}.\mathbf{l})\exp(-i\mathbf{k}'.\mathbf{l}')\int \psi_{n,\mathbf{k}}^*(\mathbf{r})\psi_{n,\mathbf{k}'}(\mathbf{r})\,d\mathbf{r} \tag{7}$$

Since Bloch functions belonging to different wave-vectors are orthogonal, we have

$$\int a_n{}^*(\mathbf{r}-\mathbf{l})a_n(\mathbf{r}-\mathbf{l}')\,d\mathbf{r} = \frac{1}{N}\sum_{\mathbf{k}}\exp[i\mathbf{k}.(\mathbf{l}-\mathbf{l}')]$$

$$= \delta_{\mathbf{l}\mathbf{l}'} \tag{8}$$

Hence Wannier functions on adjacent sites are orthogonal.

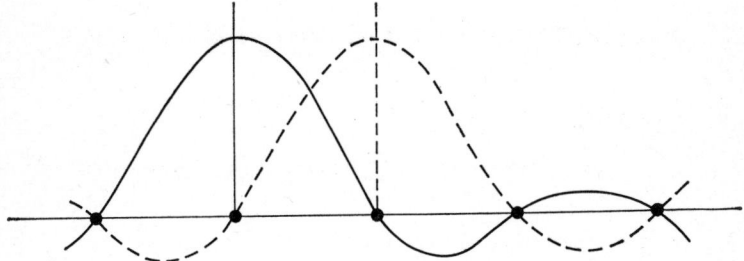

FIG. 1. Wannier functions on adjacent lattice sites.

We want a solution of the Schroedinger equation for an electron moving in the potential of an isolated impurity atom in an otherwise perfect crystal lattice, i.e. we want solutions of

$$(\mathscr{H}_0 + \mathscr{U})\chi = E\chi \tag{9}$$

We will try to construct a solution in which an envelope function is superimposed on localized functions centred on lattice sites, and assume

$$\chi(\mathbf{r}) = \sum_{n,\mathbf{l}} F_n(\mathbf{l})a_n(\mathbf{r}-\mathbf{l}) \tag{10}$$

At this stage we will assume that the impurity potential is not a sharp enough perturbation to cause inter-band transitions. This means that the donor electron can be described by Wannier functions chosen from one band only, and the band index can be dropped.

The impurity potential $\mathscr{U}$ varies little over a volume of many unit cells (when not too close to the impurity nucleus itself) and so we are interested in the value of χ averaged over many cells. In

10

this situation we find that we can replace the coefficients $F(\mathbf{l})$ by a continuous function $F(\mathbf{r})$.

If we substitute (10) in (9), multiply through by $a^*(\mathbf{r}-\mathbf{l}')$ and integrate over the whole crystal we obtain:

$$\sum_{\mathbf{l}} \int a^*(\mathbf{r}-\mathbf{l}')(\mathcal{H}_0+\mathcal{U})a(\mathbf{r}-\mathbf{l})F(\mathbf{l})\,d\mathbf{r} = \sum_{\mathbf{l}} E \int a^*(\mathbf{r}-\mathbf{l}')a(\mathbf{r}-\mathbf{l})F(\mathbf{l})\,d\mathbf{r}$$

Because of the orthogonality relation (8) this reduces to

$$\sum_{\mathbf{l}} \int [a^*(\mathbf{r}-\mathbf{l}')\mathcal{H}_0 a(\mathbf{r}-\mathbf{l}) + a^*(\mathbf{r}-\mathbf{l}')\mathcal{U}a(\mathbf{r}-\mathbf{l})]F(\mathbf{l})\,d\mathbf{r} = EF(\mathbf{l}') \tag{11}$$

Now using (4) we have

$$\mathcal{H}_0 a(\mathbf{r}-\mathbf{l}) = \frac{1}{\sqrt{N}} \sum_{\mathbf{k}} \exp(i\mathbf{k}.\mathbf{l})\mathcal{H}_0 \psi_{\mathbf{k}}(\mathbf{r}) \tag{12}$$

and also, for a perfect crystal,

$$\mathcal{H}_0 \psi_{\mathbf{k}}(\mathbf{r}) = E(\mathbf{k})\psi_{\mathbf{k}}(\mathbf{r}) \tag{13}$$

Hence, by making use of (2) we have

$$\mathcal{H}_0 a(\mathbf{r}-\mathbf{l}) = \frac{1}{N} \sum_{\mathbf{k}} \exp(-i\mathbf{k}.\mathbf{l})E(\mathbf{k}) \sum_{\mathbf{l}'} \exp(i\mathbf{k}.\mathbf{l}')a(\mathbf{r}-\mathbf{l}') \tag{14}$$

The argument is simplified if we define the quantity $\varepsilon_{\mathbf{l}}$ through

$$\varepsilon_{\mathbf{l}} \equiv \frac{1}{N} \sum_{\mathbf{k}} E(\mathbf{k}) \exp(-i\mathbf{k}.\mathbf{l}) \tag{15}$$

then

$$\mathcal{H}_0 a(\mathbf{r}-\mathbf{l}) = \sum_{\mathbf{l}'} \varepsilon_{\mathbf{l}-\mathbf{l}'}a(\mathbf{r}-\mathbf{l}') \tag{16}$$

If we now substitute from (16) in (11) we obtain

$$\sum \int [a^*(\mathbf{r}-\mathbf{l}') \sum_{\mathbf{l}'} \varepsilon_{\mathbf{l}-\mathbf{l}'}a(\mathbf{r}-\mathbf{l}')F(\mathbf{l})$$
$$+ a^*(\mathbf{r}-\mathbf{l}')\mathcal{U}a(\mathbf{r}-\mathbf{l})F(\mathbf{l})]\,d\mathbf{r} = EF(\mathbf{l}')$$

or

$$\sum [\varepsilon_{\mathbf{l}-\mathbf{l}'} + \mathcal{U}(\mathbf{l},\mathbf{l}')]F(\mathbf{l}) = EF(\mathbf{l}') \tag{17}$$

where

$$\mathscr{U}(1, 1') \equiv \int a^*(\mathbf{r} - 1')\mathscr{U}a(\mathbf{r} - 1)\, d\mathbf{r}$$

$$= \langle a(\mathbf{r} - 1')|\mathscr{U}|a(\mathbf{r} - 1)\rangle \qquad (18)$$

in the Dirac notation.

If we replace $\mathbf{k}$ by its quantum mechanical operator equivalent $(-i\nabla)$, then $E(\mathbf{k}) = E(-i\nabla)$. Further, if we assume that $E(\mathbf{k})$ is a continuous function of $\mathbf{k}$ in a given energy band, and if $\phi(\mathbf{r})$ is any continuous function of $\mathbf{r}$, then

$$E(-i\nabla)\phi(\mathbf{r}) = \sum_1 \varepsilon_1 \exp[i(-i\nabla) \cdot 1\phi(\mathbf{r})] \qquad (19)$$

from the inverse of (15).

Thus

$$E(-i\nabla)\phi(\mathbf{r}) = \sum_1 \varepsilon_1 [1 + 1.\nabla + \tfrac{1}{2}(1 \cdot \nabla)^2 + \ldots]\phi(\mathbf{r})$$

However, the Taylor expansion of $\phi(\mathbf{r} + 1)$ is given by

$$\phi(\mathbf{r} + 1) = \phi(\mathbf{r}) + 1.\nabla\phi(\mathbf{r}) + \ldots$$

and so

$$E(-i\nabla)\phi(\mathbf{r}) = \sum_1 \varepsilon_1 \phi(\mathbf{r} + 1) \qquad (20)$$

If we substitute from (20) into (17) we obtain

$$\{[E(-i\nabla) - E]F(\mathbf{r})\}_{\mathbf{r}=1'} + \sum_1 \mathscr{U}(1, 1')F(1) = 0 \qquad (21)$$

Since $\mathscr{U}$ is assumed to vary slowly from cell to cell we have

$$\mathscr{U}(1, 1') = 0 \qquad for \qquad 1 \neq 1'$$

because of the orthogonality of Wannier functions on different lattice sites. So, replacing $\mathscr{U}(1, 1')$ by $\mathscr{U}(\mathbf{r})$, evaluated at $\mathbf{r} = 1'$ equation (21) becomes

$$[E(-i\nabla) - E]F(\mathbf{r}) + \mathscr{U}(\mathbf{r})F(\mathbf{r}) = 0 \qquad (22)$$

which is evaluated at each lattice site. Because of the widespread nature (in terms of unit cells) of $F(\mathbf{r})$, it is possible to interpolate between adjacent lattice sites and treat $F(\mathbf{r})$ as a continuous function of $\mathbf{r}$. In this way a differential equation is obtained in place of the difference equations (17).

If we normalize χ in a unit cell of volume V/N, where V is the volume of the crystal and N is the number of atoms, then

$$\chi = \left(\frac{V}{N}\right)^{1/2} \sum_{\mathbf{l}} F(\mathbf{l})a(\mathbf{r}-\mathbf{l}) \tag{23}$$

Hence the probability p of an electron, which is described by (23), being in a volume $\delta V (V \gg \delta V \gg V/N)$ is given by

$$p = \int_{\delta V} |\chi|^2 \, d\mathbf{r}$$

$$= \frac{V}{N} \int_{\delta V} \sum_{\mathbf{l}} F^*(\mathbf{l})a^*(\mathbf{r}-\mathbf{l}) \sum_{\mathbf{l}} F(\mathbf{l})a(\mathbf{r}-\mathbf{l}) \, d\mathbf{r} \tag{24}$$

Assuming that there is negligible variation in $F(\mathbf{r})$ over δV and remembering that $a(\mathbf{r}-\mathbf{l})$ falls off quickly outside the cell specified by $\mathbf{l}$, we have

$$p \simeq \frac{V}{N}|F(\mathbf{l})|^2 \int_{\delta V} \sum_{\mathbf{l},\mathbf{l}'} a^*(\mathbf{r}-\mathbf{l})a(\mathbf{r}-\mathbf{l}') \, d\mathbf{r}$$

$$= |F(\mathbf{l})|^2 \delta V \tag{25}$$

since the number of unit cells in δV is $N\delta V/V$.

So we see that the 'large scale' motion of a donor electron can be described by the envelope function $F(\mathbf{r})$ and the energy states of the donor-impurity centre are obtained by solving the so-called 'effective mass equation' (22) with $\mathscr{U} = e^2/\varepsilon r$. However, some modifications to this simple theory are necessary as indicated in Chapter 1.

Glossary

It has been impossible to avoid using one symbol for two different quantities in some instances. However, this should not cause any confusion as it should be clear from the context which meaning is relevant. A glossary of the more frequently used symbols follows.

c	Velocity of light
C_{12}, etc.	Components of the elastic tensor
D	Zero field splitting parameter
D_u	Deformation potential (conduction band)
D_v	Deformation potential (valence band)
d	Skin depth for e.m. radiation
E	Energy
E_I	Donor-impurity ionization energy
e	Electron charge
f	Natural fractional abundance of Si^{29} or Ge^{73} nuclei
g, g_h	Electron and hole g-factors respectively
$g_\parallel, g_\perp$	Components of the electron g-tensor
$\delta g_\parallel, \delta g_\perp, \delta_g$	Shifts from the free electron g-factor
$g_{C.E.}$	Conduction electron g-factor
g_e	Free electron g-factor
g_N, γ_i	Nuclear g-factor
g_0	Isotropic g-value for electrons in unstrained silicon or germanium crystals
H	Magnetic field
$2\pi\hbar, h$	Planck's constant
$h.f.s.$	Hyperfine splitting
I	Nuclear spin angular momentum in units of $\hbar$
k	Boltzmann's constant
$\mathbf{k}$	Electron wave vector
M_N	Mass of a nucleus

m_F	Magnetic quantum number corresponding to the total angular momentum of electron and nucleus
m_s, m_J	Electron magnetic quantum numbers
m_I, m_1, m_2	Nuclear magnetic quantum numbers
m_e	Free electron mass
$m_\parallel, m_\perp$	Longitudinal and transverse components of the effective-mass tensor for ellipsoidal equi-energy surfaces
m^*	A general electron effective mass
N_a	Number of acceptor-impurity atoms per cm^3
N_d	Number of donor-impurity atoms per cm^3
$\mathbf{p}$	Electron momentum
$\mathbf{q}$	Phonon wave vector
S	Mechanical strain
$\mathbf{S, L, J}$	Atomic angular momenta in units of $\hbar$
S_d	Rate of ionization of neutral donor impurities
T	Mechanical stress or temperature
T_1, T_2, T_s, T_x, T_N	Relaxation times
u	Velocity of sound in a solid
V	Crystalline potential
$\bar{V}_1, \bar{V}_2$	Velocities of longitudinal and transverse vibrations in a solid
W	Activation energy
w	Hopping frequency
β	Bohr magneton
β_N	Nuclear magneton
Δ	Magnitude of nuclear polarization
∇	'Gradient' operator
∇^2	The Laplacian operator
δ	Spin-orbit splitting of a valence band
$\delta_{ll'}$	Kronecker delta: $\delta_{ll'} = 1$, 0 for $\mathbf{l} = \mathbf{l'}$, $\mathbf{l} \neq \mathbf{l'}$ respectively
ε	Dielectric constant
Λ	Hyperfine structure anomaly
μ	Electron spin magnetic moment
μ_0	Permeability of free space
ν	Frequency
ρ	Density or resistivity

τ	Mean free time between collisions for conduction electrons
τ_l	Lifetime of an electron state
ψ, Ψ, χ	Electron wave functions
ω	Angular frequency
(110)	A crystal plane
{110}	A set of equivalent crystal planes
[111]	A direction in a crystal
$\langle 111 \rangle$	A set of equivalent crystal directions

INDEX